Prevention Specialist Exam Study Guide

The *Prevention Specialist Exam Study Guide* helps readers to understand the competencies and knowledge necessary to become a Prevention Specialist (PS) and adequately prepares prevention professionals to pass the Prevention Specialist certification exam.

With this book, Nicole Augustine aims to close the gap in existing literature for the PS exam and enhance the prevention workforce so that society is better equipped to address current and future substance misuse challenges and improve long-term health outcomes for all. Divided into six domains, each module of this study guide contains a self-assessment, suggested readings, and a review of the information covered in the PS exam. A chapter covering the overall credentialing process and the additional requirement variations by the state is included.

Substance prevention professionals around the world looking to become a credentialed professional will find this one-of-a-kind resource indispensable.

Nicole M. Augustine gained the Prevention Specialist credential in 2014 and has worked at every level of prevention practice – from providing prevention education to providing training and technical assistance to communities, states, and federal agencies. Nicole owns RIZE Consultants Inc, where her professional services include coaching professionals on how they can become certified too! She serves as an Advanced Implementation Specialist with the *Opioid Response Network* and a subject matter expert for the Prevention Technology Transfer Center network.

"The IC&RC Prevention Specialist (PS) exam is one of the most difficult exams I have taken in my academic and professional career. Other PS colleagues reported the lack of comprehensive resources to help prepare for the exam. I was privileged to be one of the first to use this Prevention Specialist Study Guide. Compared to other materials, I found this resource to include current substance use trends and prevention models in the field. By using this study guide, I was well prepared for the exam and passed it on my first attempt with a high score. It is my honor to endorse this author, Nicole Augustine, and the Prevention Specialist Study Guide."

Heather D. Sharp, *MA, CPS, Program Director,*
Madison Substance Awareness Coalition.

"In the need to increase the prevention workforce, this provides a great opportunity to ensure this happens. Nicole has knowledge about substance abuse prevention and stays grounded to the field. This guide will provide the opportunity for individuals to learn the key steps in prevention. I am sure if you utilize this guide, your professional prevention knowledge will increase."

Mr Tracy Johnson, *TTJ Group LLC*

"Nicole is known as one of the premier prevention specialists in North Carolina, and is an outstanding trainer and teacher, providing exceptional workshops and seminars across the state on a variety of topics. Her information is always top notch and state of the art, giving participants more than they expected!"

Debbie Caton Rogers, *Executive Director,*
NC Foundation for Alcohol and Drug Studies (NCFADS)

"While school certainly prepared me for some aspects of the workforce, others needed some clarity. As a new graduate stepping into the field of addiction, policy, and research, Nicole's book clarified some of those questions and supported me in my efforts to lead diverse fellow professionals, build community relations, and create successful interventions. My confidence in this field is much higher after reading this book, and I'd recommend any new or seasoned professional take some time to read it, too, as I assure you will leave learning something new. This book is not just for prevention specialists, it is for anyone with a passion for public health!"

Jessica, *Social Worker*

"Nicole Augustine possesses an incredibly valuable, yet often, all too rare, combination of gifts: intellectual prowess, insatiable curiosity, compassionate convictions, innovative insights, and engaging communication skills. These remarkable attributes have made Nicole one of our nation's leading, and most effective voices for innovative skills and capacity-building within the substance misuse prevention field. All of these incredible gifts are on full display in this compelling study guide. Doing what she does best, Nicole, saw a need in our prevention field, (a scarcity of practical study resources for those seeking certification in Prevention Science), and decided to apply her decade-plus experiences and subject matter expertise, to produce the best study guide I've read over my close to three-decades-long career in this profession. More importantly, the intimate, engaging, and nurturing communicative tone and style, that is the hallmark of her training and coaching success, is conveyed throughout the writing of this study guide. The reader is immediately drawn into each paragraph and chapter, as if, they are sitting with a close friend and mentor, leading and supporting them on their journey toward certification. I cannot think of a better resource for the prevention professional."

Carlton Hall, *Founder, CEO, Carlton Hall Consulting LLC*

"This study guide is a long overdue and much-needed resource to empower prevention professionals to achieve certification, which in turn supports workforce development in a field whose value has finally come to the forefront due to the pandemic's impact on behavioral health. In the nearly 20 years that I have worked as a certified prevention specialist within the U.S. prevention network at national, tribal, regional, and local levels I have seen the profession deepen its evidence base, strengthen standardized knowledge and skillsets for its workforce, and prove its effectiveness by establishing positive change in communities across the country. I have also seen the evolution of the certification exam. When I took it in the 2000s it had a heavy focus on treatment with a minor focus on prevention which resulted in approximately a 50% pass rate. Nearly two decades later the pass rate has barely increased even though the exam is now entirely prevention-focused. The ultimate strength of this study guide is that the author is a preventionist whose expertise spans both grassroots and systems-level prevention programs, making this resource helpful to any role in the prevention field. It will certainly increase the exam's pass rate and its availability is well-timed for a growing field."

Jane Goble-Clark, *MPA, CPS, CEO, Promise Resource Network*

"Nicole Augustine has written a riveting resource guide that will serve the prevention workforce well! This brilliant guide is full of important, and practical information to better prepare prevention professionals for the field, and exam. I have been in the prevention field for over 25 years, and a guide like this would have proven extremely valuable in preparing for my credentialing exam!"

Ramona Mosley, *MS, CPS, Health Equity Prevention Practitioner*

Prevention Specialist Exam Study Guide

Nicole M. Augustine

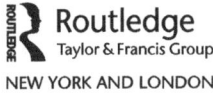
Routledge
Taylor & Francis Group

NEW YORK AND LONDON

Cover image: Getty Image

First published 2023
by Routledge
605 Third Avenue, New York, NY 10158

and by Routledge
4 Park Square, Milton Park, Abingdon, Oxon, OX14 4RN

Routledge is an imprint of the Taylor & Francis Group, an informa business

© 2023 Nicole M. Augustine

Library of Congress Cataloging-in-Publication Data
A catalog record for this title has been requested

ISBN: 978-0-367-51466-2 (hbk)
ISBN: 978-0-367-51465-5 (pbk)
ISBN: 978-1-003-05394-1 (ebk)

DOI: 10.4324/9781003053941

Typeset in Baskerville
by MPS Limited, Dehradun

I dedicate this book to my grandmother, Mrs. Genita Alice Walker (1929–2021). Thank you for raising me and helping me to build the resilience necessary to overcome my ACEs.

Additionally, I dedicate this book to our ancestors, who are the reason we're possible; the changemakers in society with big ideas for social change, and the policy advocates shedding light on social inequalities. I dedicate this book to YOU and your commitment to social progress and growth so that all of us can live a more fulfilling life.

Contents

Preface   xi
Acknowledgments   xiii

PART I
The Value of the Prevention Specialist Certification   1

1 Professionalization of the Prevention Field   3

2 The Sociocultural Context of Prevention Practice   6

PART II
**The Prevention Specialist Professional
Competencies**   13

3 Domain I: Planning and Evaluation   15

4 Domain II: Prevention Education and Service Delivery   38

5 Domain III: Communication   54

6 Domain IV: Community Organization   65

7 Domain V: Public Policy and Environmental Change   73

8 Domain VI: Professional Growth and Responsibility   81

PART III
Practice Tests and Other Resources   103

9 Preparing to Become Credentialed   105

10 Understanding the Correct Answer   121

11 Glossary of Terms   144

    Appendix A: History of Prevention Perspectives   159
    Index   161

Preface

I remember when I first set out to study for the Prevention Specialist (PS) exam. It was at the same time that I was studying for the Master Certified Health Education Specialist (MCHES) exam. I was surprised by the dearth of study materials for the PS exam and formed a study group with a few other colleagues. There were rumors that the test was challenging and many people had to take it more than once. In fact, according to the International Credentialing & Reciprocity Consortium, the PS certification exam pass rate decreased from 82% in 2016 to 62% in 2018 (IC&RC, 2019). I was very curious about this and began to do more research on the exam with the hope of discovering why current prevention professionals had difficulty passing the exam. What I found was an obvious and overwhelming need for high-quality exam preparation materials in order to improve the pass rate.

Why should we care about prevention professionals being certified?

Substance misuse causes a plethora of societal problems, many of which are preventable. The estimated yearly cost of excessive alcohol use is $249 billion, of which 72% of this cost was associated with the loss of work productivity (CDC, Excessive Drinking is Draining the US Economy, 2018). Additionally, the US life expectancy has declined, and this decline is associated with the increase in drug overdose deaths (CDC, Health, United States, 2018 – Data Finder, 2019; Haskins, 2019). An analysis from the Centers for Disease Control and Prevention (CDC) demonstrated that alcohol and drug misuse accounted for a roughly 4-month decline in life expectancy among White Americans; no other cause of death had a larger negative impact on this population (Kochanek et al., 2016). The costs associated with substance misuse problems are not just seen in the United States. A 2010 study examined the global burden of disability attributable to substance misuse problems and disorders, focusing particularly on lost ability to work and years of life lost to premature mortality (Whiteford et al., 2013). This study revealed how mental and substance use disorders accounted for 8.6 million years of life lost to premature mortality and 175.3 million years lived with disability. Additionally, mental and substance use disorders were the leading causes of years lived with disability worldwide, largely because these problems strike individuals early in their lives and can continue – especially if untreated – for long periods (Whiteford et al., 2013). The utilization of evidence-based strategies is paramount in addressing this global public health crisis. Establishing a competent prevention workforce will be critical for achieving success and improving long-term health outcomes for all.

I would be remiss if I did not also mention that a well-prepared prevention workforce is also paramount to addressing the behavioral health disparities plaguing so many communities across the country. Although the issue of disparities has been well documented for decades, there was something about the COVID-19 pandemic of 2020 that shed a spotlight on the breadth of the issue(s). This included a close examination of our field and the ways in which we can contribute to improving health equity.

Since the inception of the Prevention Specialist credential in 1994, there continue to remain scarce resources available to assist a professional in preparing for the credentialing exam. This book serves as a comprehensive guide to understanding the competencies and knowledge necessary to become a Certified Prevention Specialist. As we enhance the prevention workforce, our society is better equipped to address our current and future substance misuse challenges. There are three parts to this study guide:

- *Part I: The Value of the Prevention Specialist Certification*
- *Part II: The Prevention Specialist Professional Competencies*
- *Part III: Practice Tests and Other Resources*

My hope in writing this study guide is to provide the most comprehensive resource for anyone wishing to gain the Prevention Specialist credential.

Acknowledgments

Thank you so much for joining me on this journey of courage, audacity, and transformation. I'm excited to share my first book and want to take a moment to share the delightful story behind the creation of this book.

A special thanks to Karin Looper, who believed in me before I could even see myself. I thank Erika Patton, who connected me directly to my publisher. It was such a serendipitous event! An associate was talking about working for an academic publisher and Erika remembered hearing me talk about writing an academic text. Erika called me immediately and the connection was made. I submitted my proposal the next day!

I owe a special thanks to Heather Sharp, who was my first Prevention Specialist coaching client. We worked together for the two years it's taken me to write this book. Heather passed her test on the first try and with a high score! I'd also like to thank the following people who were of great help to me during the writing process: Jessica Garza, LaShonda Williamson-Jennings, and Donna Marie McMillan.

I also want to thank all those who contributed to the development of me as a Prevention Specialist: Gannett Health Services (Cornell University), Anuvia Prevention & Recovery Center (Charlotte, NC), North Carolina Prevention Providers Association, and North Carolina Coalition Initiative (Wake Forest University School of Medicine). I had some great teachers, mentors, colleagues, and friends along the way. Thank you for all the ways in which our conversations contributed to the creation of this book.

Last but not least, I want to thank the Editorial Board at Routledge for accepting my proposal. Prevention is an untapped market and it's such a great opportunity! Thank you for giving me creative liberty with this study guide. I hope that one day soon we can work together to bring more resources into prevention professionals' hands.

–Nicole M. Augustine

Part I

The Value of the Prevention Specialist Certification

1 Professionalization of the Prevention Field

The prevention field is an often unrecognized and undervalued part of our approach to health and wellness. We are a reactionary society that focuses most of our efforts on responding to illness through the strategy of treatment. As a result of this focus, the field of prevention has lagged behind our colleagues in treatment, while also consistently receiving the smallest distribution of financial support. The field comprises a variety of treatment and prevention organizations, including state and county health departments, public school systems, religious organizations, community coalitions, and private companies. Although our field has an international credentialing body that provides guidance on certification standards, states have the ability to set their own standards concerning the requirement of the credential. The additional challenge in prevention is our lack of career pathways in which new professionals can be recruited and retained. This is in contrast with the experience of someone who wants to be a substance treatment professional.

The professionalization of the substance treatment field is clear and the financial backing of this field provides evidence that most legislators don't see the value in prevention or they think that treatment is enough. However, we need both! We need sustainable treatment options for those who are struggling with addiction as well as continued prevention efforts designed to reduce the risk of addiction. It is through prevention that we will be able to reduce the number of persons experiencing a substance use disorder.

Why Not Require Certification for All?

The prevention specialist certification is still a relatively new certification with the roots only dating back to the 1990s. Like most other fields, there were those who practiced the art of prevention well before the certification ever existed. It is important to note that because of our history of knowledge around understanding addiction, our early prevention messages were not necessarily grounded in science. Most of the early messages created were focused on using scare tactics in an effort to 'scare' people away from substance use. From mock car crashes, gruesome scenes, or auditorium speaker who share how drug use ruined their lives, these scare tactics may seem like

DOI: 10.4324/9781003053941-2

they're getting through to young people, but all the effort is for naught. The evidence shows that these scare tactics don't work in preventing substance misuse and can even backfire! These approaches were widely accepted by the field and supported by politicians, https://preventionactionalliance.org/wp-content/uploads/2020/09/fear-messages-prevention-efforts.pdf.

Despite the popularity of fear-based education, the prevention science community began to publish research on more effective strategies for creating behavior change and preventing addiction. The leaders in the prevention field realized the need to raise awareness around what it meant for prevention professionals to be scientifically based in their messaging. And although we now know that scare tactics do not work, you can still see the evidence of scare tactics used today! The continued use of such strategies is one of the main reasons why the prevention field needs to be professionalized. Through the process of certification, we can improve the knowledge base of the field as a whole, resulting in improved service delivery, while also increasing our credibility and respect for the prevention field.

What do we mean when we use the term 'professionalized?' A profession is a particular type of occupation that requires specialized education and training, perhaps even involving an academic degree for more advanced tiers of the professionsThus, to say that substance misuse prevention needs to professionalize means that it needs to be recognized as a field requiring professionals who are knowledgeable about best practices in prevention, rather than relying on what may well be unfounded assumptions potentially based on fear or personal bias.

The Benefits of Professionalization

Preventing substance misuse with evidence-based practices is effective at reducing costs associated with the individual, society, and nation's health. Reducing the costs associated with addiction is a major priority for the improving health outcomes of our society. Additionally, the causes of addiction are complex and having a theoretical understanding of that complexity is important for developing effective intervention strategies.

Currently, the field of substance misuse prevention is not professionalized, meaning there is a lack of consistency in the standards for training for practitioners and accreditation for continuing education. This is why, despite the existence of an international credentialing board that provides recommendations for professionals, each local board creates its own standards for credentialing. The result of this is a large variance in the professional capacity of the field. In order to overcome these issues and ensure that evidence-based practices remain at the forefront in preventing substance misuse, it is important to professionalize the field by implementing standards in all aspects of training and practice. This will increase confidence among professionals in what they're doing since all staff will be following standardized guidelines from accredited institutions instead of simply someone's individual experience which can be biased.

The other advantage of professionalization includes the need to standardize the level of compensation prevention specialists receive. If the field is made official through standards such as certification and/or licensure, then those who work in prevention will be entitled to proper compensation for their hard work and dedication to saving lives. This is an important consideration for how we retain talent in the field. For so many prevention professionals, their job has no opportunity for career advancement. This reality must change if we intend to advance the field of prevention and appropriately respond to our community's substance misuse problems. If this issue resonates with you, I encourage you join with other preventionist in your region to advocate for the professionalization of our field.

2 The Sociocultural Context of Prevention Practice

I thought it important to use the first section of the book to lay the foundation for the sociocultural context in which we do our work. I am a sociologist, which means I'm fascinated by human interactions, community, and social norms. Early in my career, I was intrigued by how substance use patterns were influenced by cultural and social norms. Substance use is often centered around human interactions and social gatherings, and so I found it very helpful to explore this context when analyzing the community need assessment data. The data on the impact of addiction on our society is clear. The accumulated costs to the individual, the family, and the community are staggering and arise as a consequence of many direct and indirect effects, including compromised physical and mental health, increased spread of infectious disease, loss of productivity, reduced quality of life, increased crime and violence, increased motor vehicle crashes, abuse and neglect of children, and health care costs (U.S. Department of Health and Human Services (HHS), 2016). Substance misuse and substance use disorders also have serious economic consequences, costing more than $400 billion annually in crime, health, and lost productivity (U.S. Department of Health and Human Services (HHS), 2016). Alcohol misuse and alcohol use disorders alone cost the United States approximately $249 billion in lost productivity, health care expenses, law enforcement, and other criminal justice costs (U.S. Department of Health and Human Services (HHS), 2016).

Prevention has a major role to play in reducing the burden of addiction on our society. People may drink or use drugs to cope with the effects of poverty, discrimination, or trauma. Prevention empowers people in communities to address these problems together. Prevention professionals must be equipped to discuss all substances (such as alcohol, marijuana, opioids) and all behaviors (injection drug use, sexual transmission of HIV). Prevention is about developing personal competence through education and training; fostering community support; building professional networks; participating in prevention efforts at local, regional, state/provincial, national, and international levels; and making service linkages. Ethical values are central to the integrity of our profession. As prevention practitioners, we will advise policymakers on evidence-based practices that can best advance health promotion efforts. Our potential for social impact is great!

DOI: 10.4324/9781003053941-3

Let this chapter serve as the precursor to the knowledge you will gain in Part II of this book. History and context matter, and it is through the exploration of our history that we are able to better understand the complex issues surrounding the burden of addiction on our society. This chapter specifically discusses the following:

- History of US drug policies
- Stigma of drug use
- Social determinants of health
- The connection between social justice and prevention practice.

History of US Drug Policies

The United States has had a long history of drug prohibition. For as long as substance has existed, there has been a need to provide guidance to the public on safe and responsible use. The first temperance movement began in the early 1800s in response to dramatic increases in the production and consumption of alcoholic beverages. The American Society of Temperance, created in 1826 by clergymen, was charged with spreading the message of not drinking. This first temperance movement was quite successful in reducing the consumption of distilled spirits. The second temperance wave occurred in the late 1800s and was known as the Women's Christian Temperance Movement. The Women's Christian Temperance Movement played a huge part in establishing the Prohibition era of the 1920s. Although, Prohibition was successful in reducing per capita consumption and some problems related to drinking, the social turmoil it produced resulted in its repeal in 1933.

During the late 1800s and early 1900s, Americans began using drugs such as cannabis, cocaine, opiates, and other narcotics. The negative effects of these drugs on health and society were very visible. Remember this was a time in human existence when knew less about various substances and how they affected the brain and body. In fact, during this point in history, we limited knowledge about addiction. Much of our understanding of addiction was based on religion, morality, and willpower. The disease model of addiction was not introduced until the middle of the twentieth century and was in competition with widespread social philosophy of morality and racism as the reason for addiction. Because of our limited knowledge, we placed fear and negative stigmas on drugs and drug users.

Two main outcomes resulted from the drug policies of the early 1900s: the criminalizing of people who use drugs and stereotype of race and drug use. When reviewing the history of drug use and policies in the United States, it is also important to remember how the history of racism has played a role in our social response to substance misuse issues. The first anti-opium and cocaine laws were directed at Chinese immigrants in the late 1800s. In 1910, there were two major racial groups being targeted for different types of drugs: black men from Southern states were arrested for possession, while Mexican migrants living along borderlines faced arrests just because police suspected them to be involved marijuana trade even before legalization. The passing of the Harrison Narcotics Tax Act of 1914, which lead to the control and taxation of opiates and coca leaf, was just the beginning of a series of policies that attempted to control drug use in America, while inherently discriminating against non-White citizens.

Today's drug policy is still haunted by the discrimination displayed in our past. Many people would say that the current policy of 'war on drugs' was influenced by Nixon's fear-based election campaign which used race to push for anti-drug legislation. President Nixon declared that drug use was 'public enemy number one,' launching our nation into what some call an addiction war; US citizens were now facing imprisonment for their personal decisions to partake in recreational drugs. This sociocultural context became the foundation on which we have built many of our social responses to the 'drug crisis' affecting certain populations in the United States. This history matters and is important to consider when working with communities to address the disparities created by the complex environmental conditions.

Regardless of political affiliation, the War on Drugs has failed to reduce illicit drug use because it focuses on eradication and incarceration rather than education, wellness, access to care, safety, and inspiration. We have treated a behavioral health issue as a criminal justice problem, and the criminal justice system has systemically provided privilege for White citizens and discriminated against non-White citizens. In Michelle Alexander's (2020) book, *The New Jim Crow*, she details how institutional racism has resulted in the mass incarceration for people of color. She provides an example directly related to our field and clearly shows the influence of social injustice on social outcomes. Alexander writes about a study done by the Center For Law And Justice that states, while approximately 85% of the people who use, buy, and sell illegal drugs in the United States are White, 75% of those in jail or prison for drug-related crimes are people of color. White privilege is the root cause of racial inequity in America. When it comes to drug crimes, White people are more likely than others and get away with less punishment if convicted and least likely to be searched for drugs without probable just cause or reasonable suspicion. The disproportionate interaction of communities of color with the judicial system sets up a domino effect of other risk factors for the individual, their family, and ultimately their community. So why does all this matter? How does this affect prevention practice?

The criminalization of drug use has not benefited anyone. Substance use disorders are a preventable behavioral health issue, and until we focus on the prevention of such health issues we won't see a decrease in the burden of addiction on our society. As many of you know, we can arrest our way through the addiction crisis. Prevention science is based on identifying the risk and protective factors causing substance use disorders. When we conduct a thorough community needs assessment, we gather data across the entire spectrum of the community experience: individual, family, community, organization, society, etc. It is with this information that we are able to identify communities that have been disproportionately affected by structural inequality.

Stigma of Drug Use

Substance use disorders have a long history of being framed as a moral, personality, character shortcoming. Consider how the language we use to describe a person with a substance use disorder. We use words like 'dirty' to describe a urine sample or not 'clean' to describe when the person is 'abusing' a substance. And furthermore when a person is struggling to get well, we often address their behavioral health issue by incarceration. This is in stark contrast to how we respond to a person suffering from other chronic conditions.

Stigma is a learned social phenomenon that affects us all. Stigma prevents folx from seeking treatment early or ever. Of the 23 million Americans who meet the criteria for a substance use disorder each year, only 10% access treatment, and stigma is a major barrier to seeking help (Substance Abuse and Mental Health Services Administration, 2013). We as a society hold a narrative that treatment is reserved for 'addicts.' We then define 'addict' as someone who is weak-willed, lacks morals, can't hold a job, is homeless, is poor, or has any laundry list of negative outcomes we have type-casted to the word 'addict.' This picture inherently becomes the definition of when to seek treatment. As a result, many ignore early signs of risks and may be far advanced into the addiction process before they ever receive treatment.

A World Health Organization study of the 18 most stigmatized social problems (including criminal behavior) in 14 countries found that drug addiction was ranked number 1, and alcohol addiction was ranked number 4 (Kelly et al., 2010). The stigma surrounding substance use disorders is of great concern because is it a part of the sociocultural context in which we do our work. We are a part of society and have ourselves been subject to the influence of stigma in our professional practice. As we embrace the science of prevention and the science of addiction, we have an important role in lifting the veil of stigma from substance use disorders.

Our best first strategy is to adopt a new language and to be mindful of the words we use in every setting, whether professional or social. Check out the resource from Shatter Proof to learn more about person-centered language. This shift in language requires all of us working together. It is likely that you will find organizations and professionals who are behind the times or actively working to update their language. You may remember the wave of organizations removing the word 'abuse' from their agency name. While writing this book, I made an intentional effort to use nonstigmatizing language. I have also made note to bring your attention to areas where our field is still working to improve our language. Here is a list of suggested terms we can use to help destigmatize substance use disorders (Table 2.1):

Table 2.1 Examples of Person-First Language

Instead of this…	…Say this
Addict, junkie, crackhead, user, abuser, pill-popper, alcoholic	Person with a substance use disorder (SUD), person with addiction, person who uses drugs
Abuse	Risky or unhealthy alcohol/drug use, misuse (for prescriptions used other than prescribed)
Medication-assisted treatment (MAT), replacement therapy, substitution therapy	Medication for addiction treatment (MAT), medication for substance use disorder, treatment, opioid agonist therapy, medication for addiction, medication for opioid use disorder (MOUD)
Recovering addict, clean	Addiction survivor, person in remission/recovery, person not drinking or using drugs, person not currently/actively using alcohol or drugs
Addicted baby, crack baby	Infant born with neonatal opioid withdrawal syndrome (NOWS), newborn exposed to substances, baby born to parents who used substances during pregnancy.
Relapse	Reoccurrence of a SUD

Social Determinants of Health

Living in the United States, the world's wealthiest nation, should come with certain expectations such as access to quality physical and mental health care regardless of income or social status. However, there is a large gap between those who have privilege and those who do not. Many factors contribute to this gap including economic opportunities, education attainment levels, housing conditions, and employment rates. In addition, there are structural and institutional systems that perpetuate disparities, and the existence of these disparities should be considered when developing prevention initiatives.

The social determinants of health (SDOH) refer to the conditions in which people are born, grow, live, work, and age. These circumstances are shaped by the distribution of money, power, and resources at global and local levels. They include employment and occupation; class; education; early childhood development; gender roles; living arrangements; family situation and social relationships and support networks. The SDOH impact on a person's overall health status includes their risk for substance use disorder. There are five domains of SDOH (U.S. Department of Health and Human Services, 2021):

- **Economic Stability** – the connection between financial resources and health. This includes examining, poverty, employment, food security, and housing stability

- **Education Access and Quality** – the connection between education and health. This includes a focus on the quality of education, enrollment, retention and educational attainment, and literacy.
- **Health Care Access and Quality** – the connection between access and quality services to health outcomes. This includes identifying access to insurance coverage, primary, and behavioral services.
- **Neighborhood and Build Environment** – the connection between the physical environment and overall well-being. This includes examining a community's quality of air, water, food, transportation, and the safety of the neighborhood.
- **Social and Community Context** – the connection between social and community connection and overall well-being. This includes evaluating the sense of belongingness, civic engagement, social inequalities, etc.

The five domains are comprehensive in scope and provide a wonderful framework for developing prevention initiatives that are responsive to the complex issues described in this chapter. As the science of prevention continues to evolve, we will be called to leverage strategic partnerships and create change across all five domains of the Social Determinants of Health.

The Connection between Social Justice and Prevention Practice

As we recognize the role of prevention specialists in creating healthy communities, the connection with social justice becomes more evident. In fact, the lines between social justice and substance misuse prevention may be blurred, to enhance our impact on health outcomes.

Social justice is not a new concept. Social justice focuses on what happens to individuals, groups, or communities over time; the focus might be one of the power relationships (e.g., racial injustice) or one of the systems (e.g., judicial, educational, etc.). The United Nations (2006) say social justice may be broadly understood as the fair and compassionate distribution of the fruits of economic growth. The principles of social justice are rooted in concepts such as equity, participation, and empowerment. These include access to health care, discrimination based on race, socioeconomic status, or other factors that prevent full engagement in society. Social justice also includes equality in our shared responsibility to promote healthy behaviors and choices.

When we think about social justice, the conversation often centers on disparities in health outcomes by race/ethnicity or income level. But when looking at substance misuse prevention through a social justice lens, thinking about disparities in behavior is equally important. Disparities related to culture or ethnicity may exist in how substances are used (e.g., family tradition), where substances are obtained (e.g., drug trafficking routes), and the consequences of use (structural inequality). As we critically evaluate WHY disparities occur, we are compelled to address social inequalities as a part of our work to prevent substance use disorders. As you prepare for the Prevention Specialist exam, you will learn about the theoretical concepts that guide prevention practice. This knowledge base is important in helping you to pass the exam, and will be the focus of the remainder of this book.

Suggested Readings

Addiction Language Guide (2021). Shatter Proof. https://www.shatterproof.org/sites/default/files/2021-02/Stigma-AddictionLanguageGuide-v3.pdf

Kelly, J.F., Dow, S.J., & Westerhoff, C. (2010). Does our choice of substance-related terms influence perceptions of treatment need? An empirical investigation with two commonly used terms. *Journal of Drug Issues, 40*(4), 805–818. 10.1177/002204261 004000403

References

Alexander, M. (2020). *The new Jim Crow: Mass incarceration in the age of colorblindness – 10th anniversary edition* (1st ed.). New York, NY: New Press.

Kelly, J.F., Dow, S.J., & Westerhoff, C. (2010). Does our choice of substance-related terms influence perceptions of treatment need? An empirical investigation with two commonly used terms. *Journal of Drug Issues, 40*(4), 805–818. 10.1177/0022 04261004000403

Substance Abuse and Mental Health Services Administration (2013). *Results from the 2012 National Survey on Drug Use and Health: Summary of National Findings.* US Department of Health and Human Services. https://www.samhsa.gov/data/sites/default/files/NSDUHresults2012/NSDUHresults2012.pdf

U.S. Department of Health and Human Services (HHS) (2016). *Facing Addiction in America: The Surgeon General's Report on Alcohol, Drugs, and Health.* Office of the Surgeon General. https://addiction.surgeongeneral.gov/sites/default/files/surgeon-generals-report.pdf

U.S. Department of Health and Human Service (2021). *Social Determinants of Health – Healthy People 2030 | health.gov.* Health.Gov. https://health.gov/healthypeople/objectives-and-data/social-determinants-health

United Nations (2006). *Social justice in an open world.* https://www.un.org/esa/socdev/documents/ifsd/SocialJustice.pdf

Part II

The Prevention Specialist Professional Competencies

3 Domain I: Planning and Evaluation

Self-Assessment: Perceived Competency

Rate your knowledge/skill using the five-point scale (Table 3.1).
1 = Not at all knowledgeable/skilled, to 5 = Extremely knowledgeable/skilled

Table 3.1 Domain I: Planning and Evaluation Accounts for 30% of the Test Questions

	1	2	3	4	5
Determine the level of community readiness for change.	☐	☐	☐	☐	☐
Identify appropriate methods to gather relevant data for prevention planning.	☐	☐	☐	☐	☐
Identify existing resources available to address the community needs.	☐	☐	☐	☐	☐
Identify gaps in resources based on the assessment of community conditions.	☐	☐	☐	☐	☐
Identify the target audience.	☐	☐	☐	☐	☐
Identify factors that place persons in the target audience at greater risk for the identified problem.	☐	☐	☐	☐	☐
Identify factors that provide protection or resilience for the target audience.	☐	☐	☐	☐	☐
Determine priorities based on a comprehensive community assessment.	☐	☐	☐	☐	☐
Develop a prevention plan based on research and theory that addresses community needs and desired outcomes.	☐	☐	☐	☐	☐
Select prevention strategies, programs, and best practices to meet the identified needs of the community.	☐	☐	☐	☐	☐
Implement a strategic planning process that results in the development and implementation of a quality strategic plan.	☐	☐	☐	☐	☐
Identify appropriate prevention program evaluation strategies.	☐	☐	☐	☐	☐

(*Continued*)

DOI: 10.4324/9781003053941-5

Table 3.1 (Continued)

	1	2	3	4	5
Administer surveys/pre/posttests at work plan activities.	☐	☐	☐	☐	☐
Conduct evaluation activities to document program fidelity.	☐	☐	☐	☐	☐
Collect evaluation documentation for process and outcome measures.	☐	☐	☐	☐	☐
Evaluate activities and identify opportunities to improve outcomes.	☐	☐	☐	☐	☐
Utilize evaluation to enhance the sustainability of prevention activities.	☐	☐	☐	☐	☐
Provide applicable workgroups with prevention information and other support to meet prevention outcomes.	☐	☐	☐	☐	☐
Incorporate cultural responsiveness into all planning and evaluation activities.	☐	☐	☐	☐	☐
Prepare and maintain reports, records, and documents pertaining to funding sources.	☐	☐	☐	☐	☐

Planning and evaluation are essential components of any successful prevention initiative and represent the largest area of expertise. Through planning, we can effectively implement community change initiatives, and through evaluation, we can draw conclusions concerning the effectiveness of these initiatives. Although there is a myriad of effective prevention program planning theories and models, this chapter is based on the seven-step model described in the recommended text (Hogan et al., 2003, pp. 42–65), which I found particularly helpful in preparing for the exam. Let us review the seven-step model:

1   Assess community readiness and mobilize for action
2   Assess community levels of risk and protective factors
3   Prioritize community issue
4   Assess community resources/capacity
5   Select community of focus
6   Apply 'guiding principles' and 'best practices'
7   Create a program logic model and evaluation plan

Step 1. Assess Community Readiness and Mobilize for Action (Edwards, 2000)

The initial and first part of Step 1 begins with *assessing community readiness*, a foundational activity that is often skipped in community work, which can result in a catastrophic failure of the intended plan during the implementation phase of a project. For if the readiness is low, the community will not support the initiatives developed, and the program will be halted in its progress. I have seen this happen so many times. In my role as a technical assistance provider, I often saw communities have their implementation plans completely derailed because they planned to implement a strategy that their community was not ready for. Think of an intervention designed to get families to properly store prescription medications in a community that sees nothing wrong with sharing medication. In this instance, the prevention program purchases and supplies lockboxes that are never used. Scenarios like this happen more often than you know. This is why *assessing community readiness* is Step 1.Nine stages of community readiness have been identified, and knowledge of these stages is an important first step in the program planning process.

Assessing Community Readiness

Community norms actively tolerate or encourage the problem behavior, as the community nor its leaders, recognize the issue as a problem, although the behavior may be expected of one group and not another (i.e., by gender, race, social class, age, etc.). The behavior, when occurring in the appropriate social context, is viewed as acceptable or as part of the community norm. 'It's just the way things are.'

Stage 2. Denial

There is little or no recognition that this might be a local problem, but there is usually some recognition by at least some members of the community that the behavior itself is, or can be, a problem. If there is some idea that it is a local problem, there is a feeling that nothing needs to be done about it locally. Community climate tends to be passive or guarded. 'We can't do anything about it.'

Stage 3. Vague Awareness

There is a general feeling among some in the community that there is a local problem and that something ought to be done about it, but there is no im- mediate motivation to do anything. There may be stories or anecdotes about the problem, but ideas about why the problem occurs and who has the problem, tend to be stereotyped and/or vague. No identifiable leadership exists, or leadership lacks energy or motivation for addressing the problem. Community climate does not serve to motivate leaders.

Stage 4. Preplanning

There is clear recognition that a local problem exists and something should be done about it. There are identifiable leaders, and there may even be a committee, but efforts are not focused or detailed just yet. There is discussion but no real planning or actions to address the problem. Community climate is beginning to acknowledge the necessity to deal with the problem.

Stage 5. Preparation

Planning is going on and focuses on practical details. There is general information about local problems and the pros and cons of prevention activities, actions, or policies, but it may not be based on formally collected data. Leadership is active and energetic. Decisions are being made about what will be done and who will do it. Resources (people, money, time, space, etc.) are being actively sought or have been committed. Community climate offers at least modest support for efforts.

Stage 6. Initiation

Enough information is available to justify efforts (activities, actions, or policies), but knowledge of risk factors is likely to be stereotyped. An activity or action has been started and is underway, but it is still viewed as a new effort, as staff is in training or has just finished training. There may be a modest involvement of community members in the efforts, and great enthusiasm among the leaders because limitations and problems have not yet been experienced. Community climate can vary, but there is usually no active resistance (except, possibly, from a small group of extremists).

Stage 7. Stabilization/Institutionalization

One or two programs or activities are running, and supported by administrators or community decision-makers. Programs, activities, or policies are viewed as stable. Staff are usually trained and experienced. There is little perceived need for change or expansion. Limitations may be known, but there is no in-depth evaluation of effectiveness, nor is there a sense that any recognized limitations suggest an immediate need for change. There may or may not be some form of routine tracking of prevalence. There is no permanent funding, but there is established funding that allows the program the opportunity to implement its action plan. Community climate generally supports what is occurring.

Stage 8. Confirmation/Expansion

There are standard efforts (activities and policies) in place, and authorities or community decision-makers support expanding or improving efforts. Community members appear comfortable in utilizing efforts. Original efforts have been evaluated and modified and new efforts are being planned or tried in order to reach more people, such as those thought to be more at risk or different demographic groups. Resources for new efforts are being sought or committed. Data on the extent of local problems are obtained regularly and efforts are made to assess risk factors and causes of the problem. Due to increased knowledge and desire for improved programs, community climate may challenge specific efforts but is fundamentally supportive.

Stage 9. Professionalization

Detailed and sophisticated knowledge of prevalence, risk factors, and causes of the problem exists. Some efforts may be aimed at general populations, while others are targeted at specific risk factors and/or high-risk groups. Highly trained staff are running programs or activities, leaders are supportive, and community involvement is high. Effective evaluation is used to test and modify programs, policies, or activities. Although the community climate is fundamentally supportive, ideally, community members should continue to hold programs accountable.

Mobilize for Action

Once a prevention specialist has assessed the level of community readiness, it might be the optimal time to *mobilize the community for action*, the second part of Step 1. Typically, community mobilization is easiest when community readiness is highest. Knowledge of the community readiness level allows you to appropriately develop a plan for mobilizing the community to address a particular problem. It is at this stage in the program planning process where a community coalition can be developed if one does not already exist. Step one is critical in gaining community buy-in and helps ensure community input in all the remaining steps. Community buy-in improves the sustainability and community ownership of prevention initiatives. Remember, our mission is to empower the community to acknowledge a problem and address it in a manner that is sustainable. If you are already practicing as a prevention professional, consider how many projects you're currently managing for which you have NOT assessed the community readiness.

For more details on how to conduct a community readiness assessment, visit the Tri-Ethnic Center for Prevention Research 2014.

Step 2. Assess Community Risk and Protective Factors

In Step 2, a prevention specialist is gaining valuable information on the community risk and protective factors, also known as the needs assessment. In prevention, we are not just interested in the current level of use or risk in a community. We are also interested in 'assessing the probability of future drug misuse within populations that are not currently using substances' (Arthur & Blitz, 2000). We also want to know what is driving the problem. Do we need interventions focused on a specific population, risk, or protective factor? This step is truly foundational to us developing the right type of response to the community substance misuse needs. A great prevention program will include community involvement and feedback from people who live in that area and know it best (community members). Ideally, if you have done step one, the community is already engaged in the prevention initiative and should be ready to be an active participant in the needs assessment step.

The information gathered from the needs assessment creates a baseline against which the final program evaluation data are compared. There are two primary activities that take place during the needs assessment:

- **Data Collection:** The gathering of information that is either archival (data that already exist) or primary (data that are created). A prevention specialist should begin the needs assessment with a thorough review of the archival data. This analysis will provide evidence of community-specific risk and protective factors. Once this is known, primary data can be collected to fill in the 'gaps' in data. Data is power, and having a great working knowledge of what's happening in your community will assist you in securing funding support for your prevention initiatives.
- **Data Analysis:** An examination of data to establish meaning and set priorities for community change. Data must tell a story. It is our job to curate the data collected and design a story that any can understand. this will help you in garnering support and communicating outcomes.

An important concept to consider is how data literacy can help us better understand and respond to the social inequalities that cause substance misuse problems. According to the Data Literacy Project (2018), 'Data literacy is the ability to access, understand, and interpret data in order to identify questions, find answers, and support decisions.' The data you gather will help you:

- Describe and define your community by demographics which include age, gender, geography, ethnic or cultural group, socioeconomic status, etc.
- Describe the consumption and consequence patterns
- Identify individual and community risk and protector factors, and
- Determine additional data needed to fully understand the substance misuse problem.

Data literacy is becoming more important in today's society because it allows everyone to be informed decision-makers. The problem with the lack of data literacy is that not everyone will be able to understand what they are seeing, thus leading them to make uninformed decisions. As prevention professionals, it is our job to stand in the gap and be able to assist communities in understanding data and then leverage that data for community advocacy initiatives.

Often our greatest challenge in conducting the community needs assessment is accessing data that has already been collected. These types of data, known as archival data, are shared through county or state-level reports.

Typically, by the time these data are released, it's at least 3–5 years old. So unless we are conducting our own community needs assessment, otherwise known as collecting primary data, we are making decisions from data that might not reflect the current issues in a particular community. This is an important consideration when creating data-driven initiatives.

As you set out to conduct a thorough needs assessment, here are some steps to improve the process:

Step 1. Define your purpose and scope
We want to begin our project by establishing our purpose and scope so we can be sure we collect all of the necessary information while doing it effectively. Ask yourself: What do I hope to accomplish with this needs assessment? Who do I need to include in my process? How will I define what success looks like at the end of this project?

Step 2. Gather the archival data
Community data that have already been collected can be a baseline for understanding current substance misuse patterns. Consider what state or county agencies you should connect with in order to get access to their data sets. If analyzing data is a new skill for you, be sure to connect with a colleague and technical assistance (TA) provider to assist you in this process.

Step 3. Decide on the need for primary data
Sometimes, we need to collect our own data. Be thoughtful and intentional in this process. If you have no experience in creating surveys or interveiw questions, seek out help from an evaluator. Be sure to be conscious of your community's literacy level or other cultural factors that could influence the development of the survey.

It's very likely that the review of the archival data will not be enough, and you will have more questions about why the data is the way it is. This will create an opportunity for you to collect your own data and begin to answer the question: 'why is this happening in my community?' You can collect primary data in a number of ways: surveys, interviews, focus groups, etc.

For more details on how to conduct a community needs assessment, visit CADCA's Assessment Primer: Describing Your Community, Collecting Data, Analyzing the Issues and Establishing a Road Map for Change 2018.

Step 3. Prioritize Community Issue

Once the needs assessment report is created, the community can then translate this information into priorities. Again it is important to have community input in the prioritization process. Their input will ensure community buy-in, engagement, and ownership during the implementation phase of the prevention intervention. Several prioritization models can guide a community through the equitable process of selecting the priority community issue(s).

Step 4. Assess Community Resources/Capacity

Resource assessments are a crucial step that is often overlooked. Not only can assessing a community's resources assist in identifying resource gaps and implementing unavailable services, but they also serve as a valuable tool for discovering strategic partners who will be in alignment with your vision for community change. This type of assessment is essential as it will later be connected to your sustainability efforts. When you have community buy-in, your partners will offer their resources to ensure the success of the program.

Step 5. Select Community of Focus

At this point in the planning process, it should be clear where the most pressing needs are in a particular community. Therefore, it now becomes important to identify the *community of focus* for your program. To accomplish this, we need to understand the Institute of Medicine's categories for target populations: *Universal, Selective, or Indicated.*

Universal

Universal prevention strategies work with all individuals in a population to prevent the misuse of alcohol, tobacco, and other drugs through education and skill-building. Think of universal prevention strategies as your most general tool, with broad application. These strategies include prevention education curricula, social media/social marketing campaigns, and any type of policy change initiatives. The mission of universal prevention is to deter the onset of substance misuse by providing all individuals with the information and skills necessary to prevent the problem. All members of the population are seen to share the same general risk for substance abuse, although risk levels may vary greatly between individuals. Universal prevention is delivered to large groups without any prior screening for risk. The entire population is assessed as capable of benefiting from prevention.

Selective

Based on their higher-than-average risk of substance misuse, subsets of the total population are targeted through selective prevention strategies. This higher-than-average risk is based on identifying known risk factors associated with substance misuse issues. This is not a diagnostic activity. The selective prevention strategy is presented to an entire subgroup because the subgroup as a whole is at higher risk for substance abuse than the general population (i.e., children of incarcerated parents or youth who are failing in school).

Indicated

For individuals who do not meet DSM-IV criteria for addiction, and yet are displaying warning signs, the indicated prevention strategy is designed to assist them. These strategies are sometimes referred to as diversion programs. It is important to remember that strategies in this category are NOT treatment. It is beyond the scope of a prevention professional to provide treatment. If there's ever a concern that someone requires treatment, it is then the ethical duty of the prevention professional to refer this person for an assessment. As prevention professionals, we are only authorized to provide screenings, which assist us in identifying those at risk for a substance use disorder, and then refer those persons on for an assessment by a treatment professional.

Step 6. Apply 'Guiding Principles' and 'Best Practices'

At this point in the planning process, the prevention professional is ready to identify the best strategy for addressing the identified needs. It is very important to remember that prevention is based on science, and so the professionals should always look first at the evidence and choose a strategy that shows effectiveness. The National Institute on Drug Abuse (NIDA) has outlined a set of prevention guidelines for developing and implementing evidence-based strategies. These strategies can be thought of in three areas: risk and protective factors, prevention planning, and prevention program delivery (NIDA, 2020). Let's review these principles.

Risk and Protective Factors

- Designed to enhance protective factors and move toward reversing or reducing known risk factors.
- Include all forms of substance misuse, including the use of tobacco, alcohol, marijuana, and inhalants.
- Focus on skills to resist drugs when offered, strengthen personal commitments against drug use, and increase social competency, in conjunction with reinforcing attitudes against drug use.
- The higher the level of risk of the target population, the more intense the prevention efforts must and the earlier it must begin.

Prevention Planning

- Schools offer opportunities to reach all populations and serve as important settings for specific subpopulations at risk of substance misuse.
- Intervention strategies would begin as early as preschool.
- Adolescence programs should use interactive methods, such as peer discussion groups, rather than didactic teaching techniques alone.
- Include a parent or caregiver component that reinforces what the children are learning and opens opportunities for family discussions about the use of legal and illegal substances and family policies about their use.

- Family-focused prevention efforts have a greater impact than do strategies to focus on parents only or children only.
- Youth programs should be long-term, over the school career, with repeat interventions to reinforce the original prevention goals.
- When selecting a new program/strategy to implement, it is important to review new programs/strategies to ensure evidence of their effectiveness.

Prevention Program Delivery

- Community programs need to strengthen norms against drug use, including the family, the school, and the community.
- Additionally, community programs are significantly enhanced when they include media campaigns and policy changes.
- Prevention programming should be adapted to address this specific nature of the substance-misuse problem in the local community.
- Programs and services should be age-specific, developmentally appropriate, and culturally sensitive.
- Effective prevention programs are cost-effective. For every dollar spent on drug use prevention, communities can save about ten dollars in cost for substance-misuse treatment and counseling.

This comprehensive list provides guidance for us in creating intervention strategies that address the identified needs discovered in the needs assessment and earlier steps of the planning process. In Chapter 2, we will discuss other considerations for implementing best practices such as cultural adaptation and program fidelity.

Step 7. Create Program Logic Model and Evaluation Plan

The final step in the planning process is developing the *logic model* and *evaluation plan*. The logic model is your roadmap for understanding how the program problem connects to the program activities, which you are using to predict the program outcomes. In community work, we are often tempted to jump straight into action, which is one of the most critical failures of most prevention programs. The logic model 'helps build understanding, if not consensus, about what the program is, what it is expected to do, and what measures of success will be used' (Hogan et al., 2003, p. 211). The evaluation plan is directly connected to the logic model, and when done correctly, will provide you with both process and outcome evaluation metrics. We will discuss the evaluation in more detail in the next section. Table 3.2 provides an example of how to create a logic model. We will build on this example throughout this chapter.

Table 3.2 Logic Model Example

	I. Logic Model	II. Evaluation Questions	III. Design and Methods
A. Goals	Reduce the number of teens reporting drinking alcohol in the past 30 days		
B. Strategies	Reduce social access by increasing the perception of harm and the adoption of proper storage in the home.		
C. Target Group	Parents or caregivers who allow youth under the age of 21 to drink alcohol.		
D. If-then statement	If parents and caregivers understand the harms associated with underage drinking, they will be less likely to allow drinking at home. If parents and caregivers understand the science of addiction, they will be less likely to allow drinking at home. If parents adopted strategies for proper storage, they would limit the social access to alcohol in the home.		
E. Short-term outcomes	Parents and caregivers adopt a policy to no longer allow drinking as a 'right of passage.' Parents and caregivers properly store and monitor all alcohol in the home.		
F. Long-term outcomes	Decrease in the number of youth reporting drinking alcohol in the past 30 days. Decrease in the number of alcohol-related consequences reported by youth under the age of 21.		

Other Planning Models

This domain is the largest because planning requires the greatest amount of energy, and when done right can yield amazing results. There are a few planning models worth mentioning for you to be familiar with:

- Public Health Model (PHM)
- Strategic Prevention Framework (SPF)
- Center for Substance Abuse Prevention (CSAP) Six Strategies
- Communities that Care

Public Health Model (PHM)

This model can be illustrated by a triangle, with the three angles representing the agent, the host, and the environment (see Figure 3.1).

A public health approach requires not only an understanding of how the agent, host, and environment interact but also a plan of action for influencing all three. The agent is the catalyst causing the health problem. Examples include alcohol, vaping products, illicit drugs, prescription medications, etc. The host is the individual who is susceptible to developing a health problem as a result of interacting with the agent. And lastly, the environment is the context in which the host and the agent exist. In the case of our work, the environment is a societal climate that encourages, supports, reinforces, or sustains problematic use of drugs. Ideally, you want to plan initiatives that will influence all three areas.

Influencing the Agent

The agent in the public health model is the substance (alcohol, marijuana, nicotine, etc). Many of our strategies designed to influence the agent are focused on policies and practices that change access to those substances. These strategies will often be linked to the strategies designed to influence the environment.

Influencing the Host

Prevention professionals can reach people directly through schools, social programs, workplaces, and other groups. Efforts to reach the host are often focused on skill-building strategies or strategies to increase awareness of substance misuse issues.

Influencing the Environment

Environments include schools, families, neighborhoods, and communities, as well as the broader social and cultural environments that are influenced by

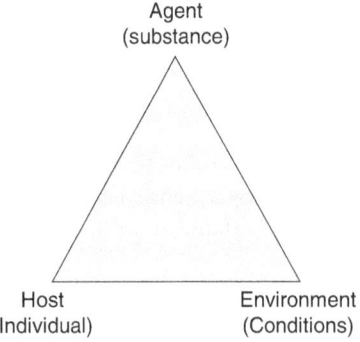

Figure 3.1 Public Health Model Triangle.

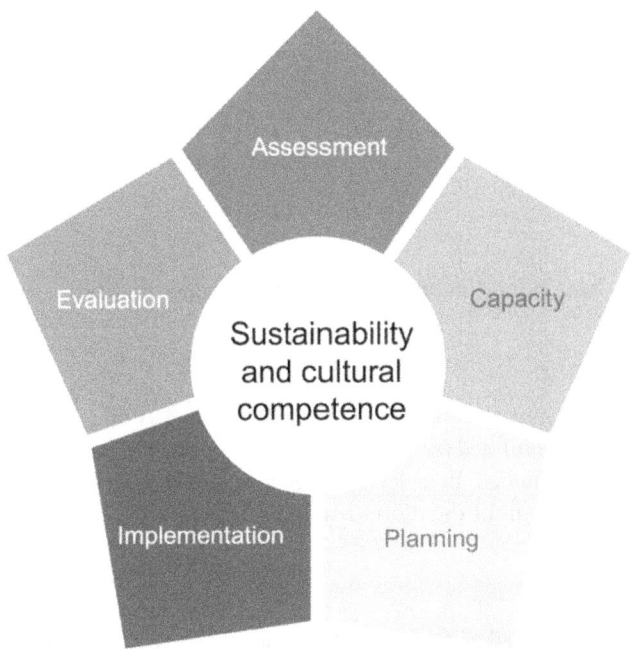

Figure 3.2 SPF Diagram of Sustainability and Cultural Competence.

legislation, pricing, advertising, and media portrayals of alcohol, tobacco, and other drug use. When we develop strategies to influence the environment, we are intentionally changing the community norms to support healthy behaviors.

Strategic Prevention Framework

The Strategic Prevention Framework (SPF) is the most commonly used planning model and was developed by the Substance Abuse and Mental Health Services Administration (*A Guide to SAMHSA's Strategic Prevention Framework*, 2019). It consists of six planning activities and two cross-cutting activities when planning prevention initiatives (Figure 3.2).

Assessment

Assess population needs, resources, and readiness to address needs and gaps.

Capacity

Mobilize and/or build capacity to address needs.

Planning

Develop a comprehensive plan.

Implementation

Implement evidence-based prevention programs and strategies.

Evaluation

Evaluate, monitor, sustain, and improve or replace strategies that fail.

Sustainability – Cross-cutting

Sustain the prevention initiative beyond the initial funding. Often in prevention, our initiatives are funded by temporary grant opportunities, designed to jumpstart community change. In order to see generational change, we must focus efforts on sustaining all of the aforementioned activities.

Cultural Competence – Cross-cutting

Conduct all prevention practice in a way that respects the culture and diversity of the community being served. In Chapter 4, I will discuss more about our movement away from the term cultural competence. This is an important concept in the advancement of our knowledge as a field. For now, this planning model uses the language of *cultural compentency* and is therefore important for you know.

Center for Substance Abuse Prevention (CSAP) Six Strategies

Many states reference the CSAP Six as a guide to how the prevention workforce should plan strategies for community change. Here are the CSAP Six Strategies:

Dissemination of Information

This strategy provides information about the nature and extent of drug use, abuse, addiction and the effects on individuals, families, and communities. It also provides information on available prevention programs and services. The dissemination of information is characterized by one-way communication from the source to the audience, with limited contact between the two. Examples include tabling at a health fair.

Prevention Education

This strategy involves two-way communication and is distinguished from merely disseminating information by the fact that it's based on an interaction between the educator and the participants. Activities under this strategy aim to affect critical life and social skills, including decision making, refusal skills, and critical analysis (i.e., media literacy). Examples include using a prevention education curriculum.

Alternative Activities

This strategy provides for the participation of target populations in activities that exclude drug use. The assumption is that because constructive and healthy activities offset the attraction to drugs, or otherwise meet the needs usually filled by drugs, then the population would avoid using drugs. This strategy has been shown to be a great supplement to other strategies and should not be used as a standalone prevention intervention. Examples include host sports of music camp for youth.

Community-Based Processes

This strategy aims to enhance the ability of the community to more effectively provide prevention and treatment services for drug misuse disorders. Activities in this strategy include organizing, planning, enhancing the efficiency and effectiveness of service implementation, building coalitions, and networking. Examples include running a coalition.

Environmental Approaches

This strategy seeks to establish or change community standards, codes, policies, practices, and attitudes, thereby influencing the incidence and prevalence of drug misuse in the general population. Examples include advocating for policies in support of state-controlled sales of distilled spirits.

Problem Identification and Referral

This strategy aims to identify those who have indulged in the illegal use of drugs in order to assess if their behavior can be reversed through education. It should be noted, however, that this strategy does not include any activity designed to determine whether an individual is in need of treatment. Examples include using Screening, Brief Intervention, and Referral to Treatment (SBIRT).

Communities That Care

The Communities That Care (CTC) model is designed marshaling community resources to address problematic behavior in adolescents. The main goal is to create a 'community prevention board' tasked with identifying the risk and protective factors and organizing the implementation of evidence-based strategies. The theoretical framework guiding this planning model is based on Hawkins and Catalano's Social Development Strategy (SDS) (Communities that Care, 2022).

The SDS is a theory that merges three major perspectives on how behavior changes over time and develops from experiences with others in social learning environments: control theory, social learning, and difference association (University of Washington School of Social Work, 2019). The Control Theory perspective sees prosocial bonding as promoting prosocial behavior, while antisocial bonding promotes antisocial behavior; Social Learning suggests behavior is learned through rewards and punishment--and Differential Association proposes there's a separate and parallel path for prosocial and antisocial behavior (University of Washington School of Social Work, 2019).

CTC has five planning stages (Communities that Care, 2022):

- **Get Started** – Identify a lead agency, key stakeholders, and staffing needs.
- **Get Organized** – Development of a community prevention board, or work with an existing coalition to galvanize support for the community change initiative.
- **Develop Community Profile** – Develop a community risk and protective factors profile. Identify community resources and identify gaps in resources needed to address community needs.
- **Create a Plan** – Develop an action plan to align the need, resources, and outcomes. For strategies for strengthening protective factors.
- **Implement and Evaluate** – Maintain fidelity to the plan created in the previous step, while also monitoring any adaptations and outcomes over time.

Program Evaluation

Program evaluation is often the most intimidating part of prevention planning. Few prevention professionals have obtained the academic background or experience needed, to understand how program evaluation should be conducted. In practice, you can hire a program evaluator to ensure that your evaluation is conducted properly. However, in preparation for the prevention specialist exam, it is important that you have a good understanding of how to conduct a sound program evaluation. Additionally, having this foundational knowledge will assist you in communicating effectively with your program evaluator and setting clear goals and objectives for your intended project.

Evaluation is the systematic collection and analysis of information gathered (data) – it is not random or haphazard. It provides information about program activities, characteristics, and outcomes; and, answers questions such as Who?, What?, How?, Why?, and So What?. Most importantly, it is used to reduce uncertainty, improve effectiveness, and ultimately, make better decisions about the prevention program/strategy being implemented. When we reflect on our work with communities, we may think of evaluation as a complex, formal, and difficult process. Many times the significance and value of evaluation are not immediately apparent to people who work to deliver the actual services, or to the people who benefit from the prevention initiative.

Evaluation provides tangible evidence that you are putting resources into prevention programs that work. Evaluation is also just as useful to determine what doesn't work in a program and provides the information you can use to improve your current efforts. If you have a prevention program that works, you should share this success with funding sources, stakeholders, residents, and the community at large. Consider the opportunity to present at conferences, publish articles, blogs, and contribute to the evidence that Prevention Works!

Conducting a program evaluation will help you improve your program. You will be able to say with confidence that changes or improvements in the program are directly related to your program's evaluated intervention(s). Evaluation should not be something that is done if you have some extra time and resources, or only when you are required to do it. Rather, evaluation is a process integral to effectiveness and should inform prevention planning and implementation.

Evaluation Terms and Concepts

Process Evaluation

Process evaluation is valuable in helping us to auto-correct early on in the implementation phase of a project, which can positively affect the outcome evaluation. Process evaluation involves analyzing how implementation activities are delivered. It covers the following:

- Who delivers the strategy, and how often?
- To what extent is the strategy implemented as planned?
- How is the intervention received by the target group and program staff?
- What are barriers to intervention delivery?
- Was the data used to make improvements/refinements? If so, what changes were made?

Outcome Evaluation

Outcome evaluation measures a program's results and helps determine whether a program or strategy produced the changes it intended to achieve. A comprehensive outcome evaluation will include:

- An assessment of the impacts of each program component
- Data from a population group
- Choices of evaluation designs – For example, assessing change before and after an intervention or comparing an intervention group to a

comparison group. Adding a comparison group or community helps you determine whether your target population would have improved over time even if it had not experienced your intervention.
* What actually worked in comparison with what you thought would work.

Outcomes or Impact

Outcomes and impact look at how the participants' lives were changed or affected by the program activities. This process includes both short-term and long-term outcome measures.

Outputs

Outputs refer to the number of opportunities the program has to create changes, such as the number of clients served and how many hours the program was in the field (Hogan et al., 2003, p. 215). Your outputs are directly connected to the process evaluation and do not provide evidence that the program is creating change. This is probably the most confusing concept for many prevention professionals. Here's a great analogy that I believe will help you understand the concept. Let's say you've decided to increase your physical activity. Your outputs will be the number of times your workout, or the amount of time you spend working out. The outcomes would be the results you experience because of the outputs (increates stamina, reduced negative health experiences, etc).

Let us revisit our sample logic model from earlier and look at the type of evaluation questions we would ask (Table 3.3).

Evaluation Methods and Study Design

The last major concept to review is *evaluation methods and study design*. Evaluation is an important component of any successful prevention initiative. Through evaluation, we can articulate the program design, implementation strategies, and outcomes. This information allows us to share our lessons learned and successes with the field while strengthening our ability to sustain our efforts.

Data Collection Options

There are two main types of data we collect: **archival** and **primary**. Archival data are existing data, while primary data represent the type of data we collect first-hand. Archival data can be critical to understanding the general scope and magnitude of a community health problem. However, archival data are often not enough, therefore, we collect additional data to help answer community-specific questions. Additionally, primary data collection is needed to evaluate the implementation activities and assess the short- and long-term outcomes of the prevention initiative. There are three main ways we collect data to assess impact: (1) posttest only, (2) pretest and posttest, and (3) pretest and posttest with a comparison group.

Table 3.3 Logic Model Example with Evaluation Questions

	Logic Model	Evaluation Questions	Design and Methods
Goals	Reduce the number of teens reporting drinking alcohol at home or with adults in the past 30 days	Was underage drinking reduced in the community?	
Strategies	Utilize information dissemination and prevention education strategies to reduce social access by increasing the perception of harm and the adoption of proper storage in the home.	What was the reach of the information dissemination campaign? How many parents and caregivers adopted a proper storage policy for their homes?	
Target Group	Parents or caregivers who allow youth under the age of 21 to drink alcohol.	How many parents and caregivers have a low perception of harm concerning underage drinking?	
If-then statement	If parents and caregivers understand the harms associated with underage drinking, they will be less likely to allow drinking at home. If parents and caregivers understand the science of addiction, they will be less likely to allow drinking at home. If parents adopted strategies for proper storage, they would limit the social access to alcohol in the home.	How many participated in the parent prevention education program? How many parents believe underage drinking is not a problem? How many participants left the prevention education experience with no change in mindset? How many parents report not properly storing alcohol in the home?	
Short-term outcomes	Parents and caregivers adopt a policy to no longer allow drinking as a 'right of passage.' Parents and caregivers properly store and monitor all alcohol in the home.	How many participants have a high perception of harm concerning underage drinking?	
Long-term outcomes	Decrease in the number of youth reporting drinking alcohol at home in the past 30 days. Decrease in the number of alcohol-related consequences reported by youth under the age of 21.	How many teens report drinking alcohol at home with adults in the last 30 days?	

Types of Data

When collecting data, we should also include a mix of **qualitative** and **quantitative** evidence. These two types of data are often confused, and a trick to remembering the difference is to look at the root of each word: quality vs. quantity. *Qualitative data* are descriptive data that provide in-depth information on the subject of interest. Attaining this information is primarily accomplished by asking open-ended questions. Although these types of data are informative, it is typically not generalizable, as it represents a small perspective of few people. Alternatively, *quantitative data* are focused on describing an issue numerically. Often folx will use quantitative data to make generalized statements about the overall population, however, this can only be done when a representative sample of data has been collected. A representative sample must reflect the characteristics of the larger population.

Evaluation Methods

Evaluation methods describe how evaluation is carried out, and include the following types of methods:

- Surveys or questionnaires
- Interviews
- Tests and Assessments
- Observations
- Focus Groups
- Case Studies
- Document and Program Record Reviews
- Archival (existing) or Primary (original survey) Data

Let us revisit our sample logic model from earlier and add more details on the evaluation design and methods we would use (Table 3.4).

Table 3.4 Logic Model Example with Design Methods

	Logic Model	*Evaluation Questions*	*Design and Methods*
Goals	Reduce the number of teens reporting drinking alcohol at home or with adults in the past 30 days	Was underage drinking reduced in the community?	Community needs assessment survey
Strategies	Utilize information dissemination and prevention education strategies to reduce social access by increasing the	What was the reach of the information dissemination campaign? How many parents and caregivers adopted a	Program records Pre/post-survey design

(Continued)

Table 3.4 (Continued)

	Logic Model	Evaluation Questions	Design and Methods
	perception of harm and the adoption of proper storage in the home.	proper storage policy for their homes?	
Target Group	Parents or caregivers who allow youth under the age of 21 to drink alcohol.	How many parents and caregivers have a low perception of harm concerning underage drinking?	Program records Pre/post-survey
If-then statement	If parents and caregivers understand the harms associated with underage drinking, they will be less likely to allow drinking at home. If parents and caregivers understand the science of addiction, they will be less likely to allow drinking at home. If parents adopted strategies for proper storage, they would limit the social access to alcohol in the home.	How many participated in the parent prevention education program? How many parents believe underage drinking is not a problem? How many participants left the prevention education experience with no change in mindset? How many parents report not properly storing alcohol in the home?	Program records Pre/post-survey design
Short-term outcomes	Parents and caregivers adopt a policy to no longer allow drinking as a 'right of passage.' Parents and caregivers properly store and monitor all alcohol in the home.	How many participants have a high perception of harm concerning underage drinking?	Pre/post-survey design
Long-term outcomes	Decrease in the number of youth reporting drinking alcohol at home in the past 30 days. Decrease in the number of alcohol-related consequences reported by youth under the age of 21.	How many teens report drinking alcohol at home with adults in the last 30 days?	Pre/post survey design Community needs assessment survey data 3 years after the program begins.

Program planning and evaluation are the foundation of our work. You are encouraged to read Chapters 3 and 8, in the Hogan et al. text for a more in-depth look into this content.

Suggested Reading

A Guide to SAMHSA's Strategic Prevention Framework. (2019, June). Substance Abuse and Mental Health Services Administration. https://www.samhsa.gov/sites/default/files/20190620-samhsa-strategic-prevention-framework-guide.pdf

Assessment Primer: Describing Your Community, Collecting Data, Analyzing the Issues and Establishing a Road Map for Change. (2018). https://www.cadca.org/resources/assessment-primer-describing-your-community-collecting-data-analyzing-issues-and

Evaluation Primer: Setting the Context for a Drug-Free Communities Coalition Evaluation. (2010). http://mail.cadca.org/resources/detail/evaluation-primer

Hogan, J., Gabrielsen, K., Luna, N., & Grothaus, D. (2003). Prevention program planning. In *Substance abuse prevention: The intersection of science and practice* (1st ed., pp. 42–67). Pearson.

Hogan, J., Gabrielsen, K., Luna, N., & Grothaus, D., et al. (2003). The logic model and evaluation. In *Substance abuse prevention: The intersection of science and practice* (1st ed., pp. 210–232). Pearson.

Planning primer: Developing a theory of change, logic models and strategic and action plans. (2018). https://www.cadca.org/resources/planning-primer-developing-theory-change-logic-models-and-strategic-and-action-plans

Selecting Best-Fit Programs and Practices: Guidance for Substance Misuse Prevention Professionals. (2018). https://www.samhsa.gov/sites/default/files/ebp_prevention_guidance_document_241.pdf

References

Arthur, M.B. & Blitz, C. (2000). Bridging the gap between science and practice in drug misuse prevention through needs assessment and strategic community planning. *Journal of Community Psychology*, *28*(3), 241–255. 10.1002/(SICI)1520-6629(200005)28:3<241::AID-JCOP2>3.0.CO;2-X

Edwards, R.J.-T. (2000). Community readiness: Research to practice. *Journal of Community Psychology*, 291–307.

EMT Associates, Inc. (2012). Studying for success: Preparing for and passing the IC&RC prevention specialist exam. https://www.pacertboard.org/sites/default/files/Preventin_Study_Guide_FINAL.pdf

Hawkins, J.C. (1992). Risk and protective factors for alcohol and other drug problems in adolescence and early adulthood: Implications for substance abuse prevention. *Psychological Bulletin*, 64–105.

Hogan, J., Grabielson, K., Luna, N., & Grothaus, D. (2003). Prevention program planning. In *Substance abuse prevention: The intersection of science and practice* (pp. 42–67). Boston: Pearson Education, Inc.

NIDA. 2020, June 10. Prevention principles. Retrieved on November 29, 2021, from https://www.drugabuse.gov/publications/preventing-drug-use-among-children-adolescents/prevention-principles

The Center for Communities that Care. (2022). *The Science* behind the program. Communities That Care. https://www.communitiesthatcare.net/prevention-science/

The Data Literacy Project – Building a data-literate culture for all. (2018). Data Literacy Project. https://thedataliteracyproject.org

Tri-Ethnic Center for Prevention Research. (2014, August 1). *Community readiness model.* Retrieved from Colorado State University: https://tec.colostate.edu/communityreadiness/

University of Washington School of Social Work. (2019). *Research brief 23 – The social development strategy (May 2019).* Social Development Research Group. https://depts.washington.edu/sdrg/rb23-the-social-development-strategy-201905/

4 Domain II: Prevention Education and Service Delivery

Self-Assessment: Perceived Competency

Rate your knowledge/skill using the five-point scale (Table 4.1).
1 = Not at all knowledgeable/skilled, to 5 = Extremely knowledgeable/skilled

Table 4.1 Domain II: Prevention Education and Service Delivery accounts for 15% of the Test Questions

	1	2	3	4	5
Coordinate prevention activities.	☐	☐	☐	☐	☐
Implement prevention education and skill development activities appropriate for the target audience.	☐	☐	☐	☐	☐
Provide prevention education and skill development programs that contain accurate, relevant, and timely content.	☐	☐	☐	☐	☐
Maintain program fidelity when implementing evidence-based practices.	☐	☐	☐	☐	☐
Serve as a resource to community members and organizations regarding prevention strategies and best practices.	☐	☐	☐	☐	☐

This particular domain focuses primarily on the implementation of prevention curricula. This chapter includes information on cultural competency, program fidelity, commonly misused substances, and the models of addiction. The theoretical frameworks responsible for prevention education curricula are discussed in Chapter 7.

Cultural Competency

Cultural competency is a critical concept in our work and is defined as the ability to serve individuals and communities in ways that demonstrate understanding, caring, and valuing the unique characteristics of those served,

DOI: 10.4324/9781003053941-6

including the cultural differences and similarities within, among, and between groups. However, we know culture is ever-evolving, thus our learning is never done when engaging in community work. There is much debate about this term and whether it is now dated, as it implies that there is some point in time when you will have gained competence on the topic of culture. Since the development of this exam, there has been a great deal of exploration into more implicit terms, such as cultural humility, cultural intelligence, and cultural awareness. Our critical understanding of this concept will guide everything we do. There is a really great resource developed by the Prevention Technology Transfer Center's Building Health Equity & Social Justice Working Group (2021) that provides a comprehensive glossary of terms related to providing culturally responsive services.

Our relationships with others require a constant balancing act between our differences and similarities. All people everywhere share much in common. In some ways, we are more similar than different. Biologically, we are all the same species, and thus, we all have the same basic needs. We seek meaning and harmony in our lives and connectedness in our relationships. We have generations of families and traditions, heritage and history, relationships with friends and others, values that direct our lives, spirituality and beliefs, patterns and habits, hopes and dreams for ourselves and for our world.

It is important to note that the field has progressed significantly, and the term 'cultural competency' is no longer the standard. We now use terms such as cultural humility, cultural sensitivity, and cultural awareness. Cultural competence implies that there is some future arrival in knowledge and experience – as if there will be some point in time when you will have gained competence on the topic of culture. Again, we know culture to be ever-evolving. Any given community contains varied ways of thinking, believing, and acting that represent the many cultures and diverse groups that exist within that community. Although communities have unique cultural profiles, all communities are communities of diversity. Each individual within that community has multiple characteristics, and possibly multiple cultures, with which they identify, that shapes their specific experience within that community. Appreciating and understanding diversity, cultural sensitivity, and culturally appropriate prevention programming for individuals and communities is an ongoing and ever-changing process that requires continual effort and patience. The goal is to learn how to continually build our ability to learn about and use similarities and differences as *assets* in prevention work.

So often, people think cultural competency is just referring to acknowledging a person's race or ethnicity. However, **culture** is much broader than that. 'Culture' can be *defined as the transfer of knowledge, experience, values, beliefs, ideas, attitudes, skills, tastes, and techniques that are shared and passed along from one member of the community to another member of the community.* Language is a major transmitter of culture. Carriers of culture include families, religious organizations, peer groups, neighbors, and social groups.

There are actually two types of cultures: **surface culture** and **deep culture**. *Surface culture* includes characteristics such as race or ethnicity, which can be seen by simply looking at someone; while *deep culture* includes characteristics that cannot be seen by just looking at someone such as values or belief systems. Many of you have heard of the iceberg analogy: *most of our identity lives below the surface and is rarely seen without further discovery or provocation.*

Continuous interplay between individuals, their perceptions, attitudes, assumptions, and behaviors, and their environment and social institutions creates dynamically evolving cultures and subcultures, where the whole is more than the sum of its parts. That is, groups are bound together by the interactions of their members, as well as by their similarities to each other and differences from other groups.

Cultural competency is a critical aspect of public health practice and is more than just understanding your community's culture. Culture is not static; it is constantly changing in response to the internal interaction of its members, between the members and different cultural groups, and to the needs and threats experienced by group members. In addition, an individual can be identified in a number of ways that are independent of each other. This enables a person to participate in more than one culture, simultaneously. Even *you* belong to multiple cultural groups, and that truth is the same for the communities you serve.

Although cultural competency is now considered a dated term, there are still lessons to be learned on how to move toward becoming more culturally competent:

1   Assess personal cultural values while acknowledging the existence of a 'cultural lens' that shapes one's interpretation of the world.
2   Become aware of the various cultures that exist within your community and abroad.
3   Understand the dynamics that may occur when members of different cultures interact.

It is important for everyone – not just professionals working with clients or communities – to be culturally competent because it allows us to better serve people. Given its importance, this section is going to outline four critical steps for working with the community to foster positive changes in behavior (Hogan et al., 2003a, p. 111):

1   Gather information from resources outside the community that helps to describe the community: relevant historical issues; current social, economic, and political concerns; traditional or culture-specific issues; languages spoken; ideas about health and health practices; educational levels; formal and informal community leaders; religion and/or spirituality.
2   Gather information from within the community: ask questions, visit the community to observe and listen, talk to community members, and become involved in community events.

3   Involve the community in program planning and implementation: obtain community 'buy-in' by ensuring the program goals and objectives are something the community cares about and is a cultural fit, which increases the likelihood of the community to sustain the initiative.
4   Involve the community in program evaluation: community involvement in the evaluation process will prove accountability and breed trust, as it ensures the evaluation is accurate and culturally relevant.

Achieving Fidelity and Cultural Adaptations in Prevention

In our prevention practice, we should be able to create *cultural adaptations* while also honoring *program fidelity*, defined as *following an evidence-based program exactly as designed by its developer*. The skilled prevention professional considers the needs of a community when developing a program, which often requires cultural adaptations. The need for cultural adaptations is great and a critical step in implementing effective prevention interventions. Whenever you choose an intervention strategy, take the time to confirm the audience it was developed for and then invite your community members to assist you in identifying adaptations. Lastly, you want to follow-up with the developer concerning the planned adaptations to make sure they arenot changing core messages or content (fidelity), but rather, adjusting how the intervention is delivered in order to make it more relatable. Adaptations inculde making modifications so the content is by members of varying cultural backgrounds and/or community members who may have different language, skills, and/or literacy levels.

The first step in creating cultural adaptations is to learn more about the community you are serving. How can one begin to identify the need for an adaptation without proper knowledge of the community of focus? You will want to consult experts who know the community best and can provide you with a valuable perspective on the community. Here's where to start:

1   **Individuals and groups from the focus community:** This will often be your first contacts in the community. Through them you will learn extensively about the community in a more direct way than just reading or hearing about it. Community members can also work with you as partners and consultants to create or adapt the program to the various groups within the community. Look for leaders of community institutions like religious congregations, civil rights groups, and arts organizations. Poorly or hastily selected people can cost you the accuracy of your information, as well as the trust of the community in later program-building efforts.
2   **Helping professionals or other persons working in similar communities or with similar problems:** These people may be

found in local, regional, or national organizations (e.g., major minority health organizations or voluntary health agencies). These organizations often have accumulated relevant information based on their experience with various diverse communities throughout the country. Such people can provide you with more specific information about the problem as it is experienced by the different cultural groups. People in local organizations can also give you pointers on how to work in and with the community, sharing with you some of their own experiences (i.e., what is culturally appropriate, what does or doesn't work well, and whom you might contact in the community to begin your planning).

3   **Research:** Although you should spend most of your time in the community, it is important to devote some time to library research so that your approach in the community is an informed one. Remember that most information from these sources is likely to cover a much broader population than you intend to work with; be prepared for significant local and regional differences.

4   **Academicians:** These are the people in academic research institutions or government agencies who have done research in your areas of interest or have personal, sociological, or historical knowledge and experience with specific ethnic or subcultural groups. They can help you interpret and clarify the findings from your library search or direct you to the most recent and relevant research.

In prevention practice, we should be able to create cultural adaptations while also honoring program fidelity. Remember our work is based on science, therefore, following a program exactly how it was intended to be executed is crucial to getting the types of outcomes that create positive change in a community. However, when needed, it is further advised to contact the developer of the program regarding any desired adaptations to implement in an evidence-based program.

   Creating cultural adaptations is not easy, but it can be done with a bit of planning. Here are some key things to think about when working on creating a culturally adapted program:

•   What changes need to be made? (ie.: are there other languages in which the program should be offered)
•   Who will adapt the changes and how long does this process take?
•   How will we evaluate our efforts?
•   Does our organization have strengths that we could leverage in order to create these cultural adaptations? (i.e., additional funds to offer staff who have specialized skills)
•   Will people from the community see us as credible if they know we're adapting content for them?
•   Do we need to consult with a subject matter expert?

Understanding Substance 'Use'

Most people have used alcohol or other mind-altering substances (including caffeine and tobacco) at some point in their life. It's helpful to understand the language we use to describe the range of experiences some may have from abstinence to addiction. Let's define this range in the following ways: no use, use, misuse, and substance use disorder. 'No Use' refers to complete abstinence or never having used mind-altering substances. 'Use' refers to the ingestion of substances without experiencing negative consequences. Any substance can be 'used' according to this definition. However, the type of drug taken and the characteristics of the individual contribute to the probability of experiencing negative consequences. For example, it's illegal for minors to drink alcohol. Therefore, any use by a minor would immediately place them in the 'misuse' category. When a person experiences negative consequences from the use of alcohol or other drugs, it is defined as 'misuse.' It's important to note that misuse does not guarantee movement into addiction. What we do know is that the younger someone is when they first start use, the greater the risk of developing an addiction. It is because of this fact that our field of prevention is so important. Prevention is the one clear strategy for reducing the burden of addiction on our society.

Now, it is very possible that some of you reading this guide knows of someone who misuses substances and doesn't appear to experience negative consequences. Remember these definitions are meant to provide a simple conceptualization of 'use.' The probability of experiencing negative consequences is directly related to the frequency and level of use. If a person uses alcohol or other drugs on an occasional basis, the probability of negative consequences is far less than if one uses them on a daily basis. At the same time, you can have someone have one misuse incident and it is traumatic enough to completely change their life.

Continuum of Care

In Chapter 3, we reviewed the IOM categories of prevention audiences as a way of understanding the various levels of prevention strategies. It is also important to understand how those categories fit into the larger behavioral health field. Figure 4.1 shows the full continuum of care.

This continuum offers a comprehensive way of viewing the opportunities to intervene and address behavioral health problems. The model includes four primary components:

- **Promotion:** The goal of these strategies is to create a supportive environment for individuals. The promotion strategies reinforce the entire continuum of behavioral health services.
- **Prevention:** These efforts are delivered prior to the onset of a substance use disorder, and are designed to prevent or reduce the risk of developing

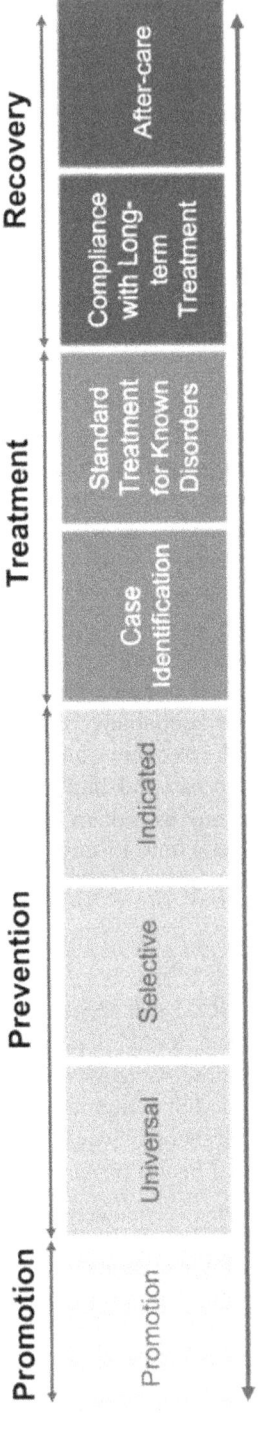

Figure 4.1 Continuum of Care Model, Promotion through Recovery.

behavioral health problems like underage alcohol use, prescription medication (such as opioids), or illicit drug use.

- **Treatment:** These services are for people diagnosed with substance use or other behavioral health disorder.
- **Recovery:** These strategies are designed to support the maintenance of wellness gained during treatment.

Although the Continuum of Care is presented in neat little boxes, it is often the experience that interventions don't necessarily fit neatly into one category or another. You will often see promotion and prevention strategies overlap, and there are even situations when prevention and recovery strategies align. Consider how the goal of prevention to prevent substance misuse and the goal of recovery to support wellness, can be strategically aligned in support of each other. Remember, there are also clear professional boundaries that exist along the Continuum of Care. Refer back to Chapter 3, and review the CSAP Six Strategies, which includes Problem Identification & Referral as a strategy we use for individuals who might benefit from a higher level of care than we are professionally competent to provide.

NOTE: Since the development of the continuum of care, there has been an evolution in our field to now include harm reduction. Harm reduction is defined as a set of practical strategies and ideas aimed at reducing negative consequences related to drug use. In theory, harm reduction approaches are not 'against' abstinence or treatment but rather acknowledge that abstinence may not be achievable or even desired by everyone. Harm reduction focuses on providing folx with the resources (which in clude eudcational resources) necessary for them to make informed decisions on reducing their harms. In the near future, we will see the formal addition of harm reduction into the Continuum of Care.

Categories of Substances

Although prevention professionals do not treat substance addiction, it is important to have a good working knowledge of categories of substances. In doing your prevention work, you will likely only provide surface-level information on the various substances. We live in the internet age, where accessing information is as easy as picking up your phone. It is very likely the youth, parents, and community members engaged will know more than you about the latest substances; and, that's ok! Your goal is not to be an expert on every substance. For this section, we will first review the five schedules of substances under the Controlled Substance Act (CSA) and then we will review the seven categories of substances.

The Controlled Substance Act

The Controlled Substance Act (CSA) is published in Title II of the Comprehensive Drug Abuse Prevention and Control act of 1970. It defines five 'Schedules' with varying qualifications for each. Drugs are tiered into their respective schedules, depending on whether they have a medical use, their potential for addiction, and safety concern(s) related to dependence liability, etc. The Act provides a system for controlling substances, adding them to schedules; and even rescheduling a substance when necessary. Petitions to add, delete or change the schedule of a drug may be initiated by any interested person, including YOU! Here's a list of the types of interested parties that can petition a change:

- the manufacturer of a drug,
- a medical society or association,
- a pharmacy association,
- a public interest group concerned with drug abuse,
- a state or local government agency,
- or an individual citizen.

When a petition is received by the DEA, the agency begins its own investigation of the drug. The DEA also may begin an investigation of a drug at any time based upon information received from law enforcement laboratories, state and local law enforcement and regulatory agencies, or other sources of information.

The CSA Schedules are as follows:

Schedule I – examples include heroin, LSD, marijuana, and methaqualone

- The drug or other substance has a high potential for dependence.
- The drug or other substance has no currently accepted medical use in treatment in the United States.
- There is a lack of accepted safety for use of the drug or other substance under medical supervision.

Schedule II – examples include morphine, phencyclidine (PCP), cocaine, methadone, and methamphetamine.

- The drug or other substance has a high potential for dependence.
- The drug or other substance has a currently accepted medical use in treatment in the United States or a currently accepted medical use with severe restrictions.
- Misuse of the drug or other substance may lead to severe psychological or physical dependence.

Schedule III – examples include anabolic steroids, codeine and hydrocodone with aspirin or Tylenol®, and some barbiturates.

- The drug or other substance has less potential for dependence than the drugs or other substances in Schedules I and II.

- The drug or other substance has a currently accepted medical use in treatment in the United States.
- Misuse of the drug or other substance may lead to moderate or low physical dependence or high psychological dependence.

Schedule IV – examples include Darvon®, Valium®, and Xanax®.

- The drug or other substance has a low potential for dependence relative to the drugs or other substances in Schedule III.
- The drug or other substance has a currently accepted medical use in treatment in the United States.
- Misuse of the drug or other substance may lead to limited physical dependence or psychological dependence relative to the drugs or other substances in Schedule III.

Schedule V – examples include cough medicines with codeine.

- The drug or other substance has a low potential for dependence relative to the drugs or other substances in Schedule IV.
- The drug or other substance has a currently accepted medical use in treatment in the United States.
- Misuse of the drug or other substances may lead to limited physical dependence or psychological dependence relative to the drugs or other substances in Schedule IV.

The Seven Categories of Substance

Society has a long history of substances and we have categorized these substances to better understand their effects. As you review these categories of substances make not how this information intersects with the CSA Schedules. It's important to note there is still much debate about how certain substances have been scheduled.

Let's review the seven categories of substances:

1   *Narcotics*

The term 'narcotic,' derived from the Greek word for 'stupor,' originally referred to a variety of substances that dulled the senses and relieved pain. Today, the term is used in a number of ways. Some individuals define narcotics as drugs related to opium, opium derivatives, and their semisynthetic substitutes, or those substances that bind at opiate receptors (cellular membrane proteins activated by substances such as heroin or morphine), while others refer to any illicit substance as a narcotic. For example, cocaine and coca leaves, which are also classified as 'narcotics' in the Controlled Substances Act (CSA), neither bind at opiate receptors, nor produce morphine-like effects and are discussed in the section on stimulants. Examples of narcotics include the following:

- Heroin
- Morphine
- Codeine, Hydrocodone
- Methadone

A note about the opioid crisis in the United States.

It is this category of substances that has received the greatest attention in the early 2000s with the advent, or onset, of the 'opioid crisis.' Interestingly, this crisis was stimulated by an increase in opioid prescriptions that were issued by doctors. This increase was due to the belief that opioids were not addictive and patients would only be given them for short-term pain relief. However, doctors themselves did not understand how addicting these drugs could be, so they gave out prescriptions with little caution or foresight. I would be remiss, if I did not mention how the role of our no pain culture and focus on customer satisfaction surveys added pressure on doctors to prescribe opioids. For many doctors, their reimbursement rates were linked to customer satisfaction, and when high ratings are linked to easing patients' pain, it became the perfect storm for the opioid crisis to brew.

As we examine the opioid crisis, it is immediately apparent that American society took a completely new approach to address this crisis today, in comparison to the response to criminalizing marijuana in the early 1900s, heroin in the 1940s and 1970s, and eventually, the crack epidemic in the 1980s. The overwhelming response was prohibition and criminalization, leading to the 'War on Drugs,' where policy action was taken to criminalize and punish those suffering from a substance use disorder. In contrast, our current opioid crisis is seen as a medical condition requiring treatment, while addiction to substances such as crack cocaine (a form of cocaine) was met with incarceration and legal consequences. If you dig even deeper you will also see that the faces of the epidemics were starkly different. The opioid crisis was largely affecting White suburban and rural communities, while marijuana, heroin, and the crack epidemic was seen in inner cities and among minority groups. As a result, the outpouring of resources to address the opioid crisis has been tremendous. This specific example has shed light on the continued structural and institutional racism in the United States, which continues to be an issue of civil rights and social justice, to which I hope we will continue to acknowledge and address.

2   *Central Nervous System (CNS) Depressants*

Depressants, also known as 'Downers,' are commonly used to reduce anxiety, induce sleep or relieve stress (Hogan et al., 2003b, p. 77). The following are examples of CNS depressants:

- Alcohol
- Sedatives
- Hypnotics
- Heroin

3   *Central Nervous System (CNS) Stimulants*

Stimulants, also known as 'Uppers' are commonly used to increase alertness and reduce fatigue. Stimulants reverse the effects of fatigue on both mental and physical tasks. Two commonly used stimulants are nicotine, found in tobacco products, and caffeine, an active ingredient in coffee, tea, some soft drinks, and many nonprescription or over-the-counter (OTC) medicines. Although the use of these products has been an accepted part of US culture, the recognition of their adverse effects has resulted in a proliferation of caffeine free products and efforts to discourage cigarette smoking. The following are examples of CNS stimulants:

* Nicotine
* Cocaine, Crack Cocaine
* Amphetamine
* Nonamphetamine Stimulants

There are a number of stimulants under the regulatory control of the CSA. Some of these controlled substances are available by prescription for legitimate medical use in the treatment of obesity, narcolepsy, and attention deficit disorders. Recent increases in the medical use of these drugs can be attributed to their use in the treatment of ADHD. With this, we have also seen situations where ADHD medications are diverted to persons who use them nonmedically (i.e., a college student taking medication to stay up and study, or an adult using to compensate for a lack of needed sleep). It is important to remember that any substance, prescription or otherwise, has the potential to be misused.

Finally, there are illicit stimulants, which are frequently taken to produce a sense of exhilaration, enhance self-esteem, improve mental and physical performance, increase activity, reduce appetite, produce prolonged wakefulness, and to just get high. As with the previous section, we can look at our policy action in the United States and encounter clear evidence of structural and institutional racism. In the United States, our drug policies created punitive distinctions between crack cocaine and powder cocaine, despite the two substances being chemically the same. The Anti-Drug Abuse Act of 1986 would assign a 100x harsher sentence for the use, possession, and/or distribution of crack cocaine, as compared to powder cocaine. The primary difference was in *who* used and/or distributed the two types of substances, and black and brown communities were more commonly associated with the use of crack cocaine. The adverse effects of this draconian law were tremendously devastating to Black, Indigenous, and People of Color (BIPOC), and we saw major surges of BIPOC disproportionately entering the US prison system, decimating families and once-thriving communities.

4   *Hallucinogens*

Hallucinogens, also known as psychedelics, can distort perception, thoughts, and mood. These substances induce illusions and hallucinations. Examples of hallucinogens include the following:

- PCP
- LSD
- Peyote
- MDMA
- Ketamine
- Psilocybin

5   *Cannabis*

Cannabis sativa L., the cannabis plant, grows wild throughout most of the tropic and temperate regions of the world. Prior to the advent of synthetic fibers, the cannabis plant was cultivated for the tough fiber of its stem. In the United States, cannabis is legitimately grown only for scientific research. *Cannabis* contains chemicals called cannabinoids that are unique to the cannabis plant. One in particular is delta-9-tetrahydrocannabinol (THC) and is believed to be responsible for most of the characteristic psychoactive effects of *Cannabis*. Be sure to familiarize yourself with the *Cannabis* policies in our country, as the tides (or, culture is) are shifting. Several states that have both medical and recreational use laws, create confusion for youth attempting to understand the harms of use on the brain and body. Primary prevention, which means no use of substances during the early stage of brain development, is our principal message. Essentially, we want the youth to delay, for as long as possible, the initiation or experimentation of ANY substance use, to the minimum age of 21.

6   *Steroids*

Steroids are commonly used to assist with a variety of medical conditions. They are typically misused by athletes who are attempting to enhance their bodies. These drugs are misused by high school, college, professional, elite, and amateur athletes in a variety of sports (ie: weight lifting, track and field, swimming, cycling, and others) to obtain a competitive advantage. Bodybuilders and fitness buffs take anabolic steroids to improve their physical appearance, and individuals in occupations requiring enhanced physical strength (i.e., body guards, night club bouncers, construction workers) are also known to misuse these drugs.

7   *Inhalants*

Inhalants are a diverse group of substances that include volatile solvents, gases, and nitrites that are sniffed, snorted, huffed, or bagged to produce intoxicating effects similar to alcohol, and when misused, create a psychoactive, mind-altering effect. These substances are found in common household products such as glues, lighter fluid, cleaning fluids, and paint products. Inhalant misuse is the deliberate inhaling or sniffing of these substances to get high. The easy accessibility, low cost, legal status, and ease of transport and concealment make inhalants one of the first substances abused by children. All inhalants have legitimate purposes of design and use, and are not to be intentionally inhaled. Preventionists shouldn't refer to inhalants as a drug, as they really are toxic and fatally poisonous when used inappropriately. Some examples of inhalants include

- Volatile Solvents – paint thinner, glue, gasoline, nail polish, markers
- Aerosol and Gases – spray paint, hair spray, liquid air duster, deodorant
- Nitrites – room deodorizer, amyl nitrite, or butyl nitrite
- Gases – butane lighter fluid, propane, helium

Models of Addiction

There is a long-standing history of addiction being viewed as a moral failing or lack of willpower on the part of the individual. Our understanding of addiction and substance use disorder has certainly grown over time. Several models have been developed to describe the addiction process. Following is a high-level overview of the various models that have existed for how we describe addiction. As you review them, you should be able to clearly recognize why stigma still remains a major barrier to our work.

Moral – emphasizes personal choice as being central in understanding why someone may develop an addiction problem, and that an individual who has developed such a problem is viewed by society as willfully violating its norms or moral code of conduct.

Temperance – developed by the Temperance movement in the 1800s and early 1900s, this model saw alcohol as a dangerous substance that caused addiction for anyone who consumed it. The temperance movement was characterized by a focus on religiosity and addiction was seen as a moral failing.

Spiritual – contends that addiction is a condition people are powerless to overcome, so they must turn their life over to a higher power and follow a spiritual path.

Education – focuses on the need for increased knowledge to reduce harm. Addiction is seen as a negative consequence people experience because they don't have accurate information about the impact and consequences of drug use.

Characterological/Personality – addiction is seen as caused by abnormalities in personality (aka the addictive personality).

Conditioning – addiction is a learned behavior in which early substance use is rewarded and thus the behavior continues to the point of addiction.

Sociocultural – substance patterns are influenced by culture, religion, family, and peers. Thus, substance use is higher among cultural groups that accept and tolerate the behavior.

Social Learning – addictive behaviors are seen as 'bad habits' that are socially learned by watching 1) what others do, 2) the situation in which the behaviors are acceptable, and 3) the positive results of the behavior.

Cognitive – focus on the individual beliefs or expectations. Using substances is mainly determined by the consequence an individual expects to receive as a result of using substances.

Biological – emphasizes the role of heredity and physiology in 'predisposing' an individual to addiction.

Psychological – substance use is secondary to another mental health concern. Substances are used to alleviate pain to deal with the symptoms of another primary mental health concern.

Dispositional Disease – addiction is a disease, making the person incapable of self-regulating their use.

General Systems – individual problematic use is seen as part of a larger 'dysfunctional' system. Often the larger system is thought of as a family. Substance use is usually a coping strategy to maintain balance in the general system.

Public Health – establishes a trifecta of the interaction between the dangerous aspects of a substance, the characteristics of the individual, and the aspects of the environment that promote substance misuse.

Biopsychosocial – some people develop substance problems because of a genetic predisposition, psychological factors, physical factors, emotional pain, environmental factors, or any combination of these.

Suggested Reading

Building Health Equity & Social Justice Working Group (2021, September). *A comprehensive culturally responsive glossary.* PTTC Network. https://pttcnetwork.org/sites/default/files/2021-12/PTTC%20A%20Comprehensive%20Culturally%20Responsive%20Glossary_Final_1.pdf

Capacity Primer: Building Membership, Structure and Leadership (2019) https://www.cadca.org/resources/capacity-primer-building-membership-structure-and-leadership

Hogan, J., Gabrielsen, K., Luna, N., & Grothaus, D. (2003a). Facts about drugs. In *Substance abuse prevention: The intersection of science and practice* (1st ed., pp. 68–99). Pearson.

Hogan, J., Gabrielsen, K., Luna, N., & Grothaus, D. (2003b). The cultural context and ethics in prevention. In *Substance abuse prevention: The intersection of science and practice* (1st ed., pp. 103–114). Pearson.

Implementation Primer: Putting Your Plan into Action (2019). https://www.cadca.org/resources/implementation-primer-putting-your-plan-action

References

Building Health Equity & Social Justice Working Group (2021, September). *A comprehensive culturally responsive glossary*. PTTC Network. https://pttcnetwork.org/sites/default/files/2021-12/PTTC%20A%20Comprehensive%20Culturally%20Responsive%20Glossary_Final_1.pdf

Hogan, J., Gabrielsen, K., Luna, N., & Grothaus, D. (2003a). The cultural context and ethics in prevention. In *Substance abuse prevention: The intersection of science and practice* (1st ed., pp. 103–114). Pearson.

Hogan, J., Gabrielsen, K., Luna, N., & Grothaus, D. (2003b). Facts about drugs. In *Substance abuse prevention: The intersection of science and practice* (1st ed., pp. 68–102). Pearson.

5   Domain III: Communication

Self-Assessment: Perceived Competency

Rate your knowledge/skill using the five-point scale (Table 5.1).

1= Not at all knowledgeable/skilled, to 5 = Extremely knowledgeable/skilled

Table 5.1 Domain III: Communication Accounts for 13% of the Test Questions

	1	2	3	4	5
Promote programs, services, and activities, and maintain good public relations.	☐	☐	☐	☐	☐
Participate in public awareness campaigns and projects relating to health promotion across the continuum of care.	☐	☐	☐	☐	☐
Identify marketing techniques for prevention programs.	☐	☐	☐	☐	☐
Apply principles of effective listening.	☐	☐	☐	☐	☐
Apply principles of public speaking.	☐	☐	☐	☐	☐
Employ effective facilitation skills.	☐	☐	☐	☐	☐
Communicate effectively with various audiences.	☐	☐	☐	☐	☐
Demonstrate interpersonal communication competency.	☐	☐	☐	☐	☐

Communication is one of the most important skills for a prevention professional. Whether you are communicating with your team, running a meeting, or delivering an engaging speech to youth about the dangers of drug use, communication is key to success. On May 2, 2013, the International Certification & Reciprocity Consortium announced the completion of a new Prevention Specialist Job Task Analysis (IC&RC, 2013). The principal result of this analysis was the development of the communication domain. Ultimately, creating a total of six performance domains instead of the historic five. Although this section is considered a new domain, it is in my opinion that no new skills are needed for understanding this performance domain. The majority of the concepts for this section were previously under Domains I (Prevention Education & Service Delivery) and III (Community Organizing).

DOI: 10.4324/9781003053941-7

Therefore, the development of this domain primarily serves as an acknowledgment of the crucial role communication plays in the prevention field. This chapter covers the following topics:

- Process Model of Communication
- Listening Effectively
- Public Speaking
- Group Facilitation
- Leadership Styles
- Media Advocacy

Process Model of Communication

Although there are several communication models, the model depicted below is most widely accepted (Hogan, 2003, pp. 233–236) (Figure 5.1).

Sender

The *sender* is responsible for sending clear messages, with the goal of improving the understanding of the receiver. This includes making sure both verbal and nonverbal communication is in sync. We will discuss public speaking skills later in this chapter and further discuss ways that senders can improve their delivery of messages to an intended audience. Theoretically, everyone is a sender at some point during a communication exchange. When we come back to this topic later in the chapter, we focus on how YOU as the prevention specialist can ensure you are sending clear messages.

Message

The *message* is the idea the sender is attempting to communicate. Although we typically think of messages as verbal, there are also nonverbal messages. For example, in the context of a coalition meeting, coalition members expect the

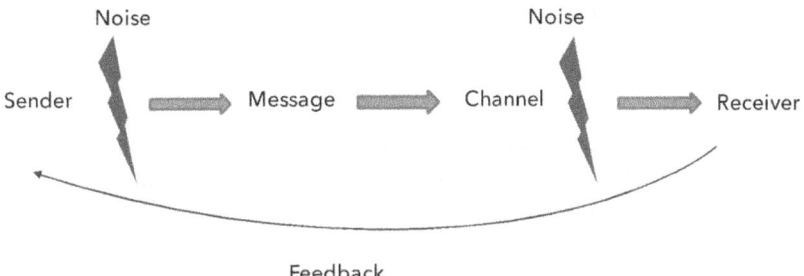

Figure 5.1 Process Model of Communication.

leader to confidently and knowledgeably provide various messages. If the coalition leader is nervous, arrives late, and appears disorganized, the nonverbal message noticeably communicates dissonance to the coalition members.

Channel

The *channel* is the method by which the message is delivered (i.e., voice, radio, television, Internet, social media, etc.).

Receiver

The *receiver* accepts the message from the sender through the channel by which it was sent. Like with the sender component of this model, everyone at some point in the communication exchange is a receiver. In the next section, we discuss the art of listening, which will assist you in listening effectively as a primary strategy to improve your prevention communications.

Feedback

Feedback describes the complex dance that occurs between the sender and receiver. This includes the verbal and nonverbal exchange that frequently places the sender and receiver into dual roles. For example, if the receiver looks confused after hearing a message, this nonverbal cue indicates to the sender that something is wrong. In this instance, the receiver becomes the sender and the sender becomes the receiver. An adept sender will notice this shift and create space to better understand the nonverbal message, before proceeding with a new message.

Noise

Noise refers to anything that interferes with the delivery of the message. This could be a number of things: noisy setting, uncomfortable setting, lack of voice projection from the sender, etc. A skilled prevention professional will plan ahead for potential noise interference and be able to quickly solve any unexpected noise interference as it occurs.

Listening

It is important to understand the difference between listening and hearing. Hearing is the physiological process of sound waves being transformed into auditory nerve impulses (Hogan, 2003, p. 236). The process of listening is not the same as hearing; it requires paying close attention to what is being said and making sense of the information that has been received. The brain is a powerful organ in the human body and is capable of processing information quickly. Your brain can understand up to 400 words per minute. However, people only speak about 125–150 words per minute (Hogan, 2003, p. 237). This gap creates space for the receiver to be distracted by noise, and loss of attention minimizes clear understanding. Listening for understanding is truly an accomplished skill, which is why it is said 'the best leaders are great listeners.' Listening requires discipline of the mind, and once you understand this concept, you can translate this knowledge into making you a better overall communicator; sender and receiver.

Information overload and noise are the biggest threats to listening. Information overload occurs when the sender has not properly considered the capacity of the receiver to take in the information provided. We've all had the experience at a conference presentation when you felt like the presenter shared so much information that you could no longer digest the knowledge being shared. Your professional development should include familiarizing yourself with the foundations of adult learning (andragogy) and basic learning principles. The problem of information overload is rarely experienced when using an evidence-based curriculum, as the curricula have been appropriately timed and segmented to fit the intended audience. Information overload is most commonly experienced in other settings such as meetings, webinars, or training.

Public Speaking

Public speaking is the most commonly used medium in our communication toolbox. Every service delivery opportunity is built upon public speaking. This is the life-blood of our work. Every prevention professional should actively seek to continuously improve their communications skills. In the previous section, I described how easy it is for the receiver to be distracted by noise. There is one type of noise to which you have control: the noise you bring as the sender. Here are some characteristics to avoid and help improve understanding when speaking.

The Moving Target

This speaker moves unnecessarily, walks, paces, or rocks to the point of distraction. Remember, movements can create 'noise' that interferes with the delivery of your message.

The Musician

This speaker fidgets and plays with keys, change, or anything that is within reach. Again, this creates 'noise' in the environment that is distracting to the receiver.

The Peacock

This speaker is nervous about how they look and is constantly tugging at clothing, fixing hair, etc. These actions communicate nervousness to the receiver and a lack of confidence. As subject matter experts, our ability to communicate with confidence is important to be seen as a trusted source of information.

The Great Scientist

This speaker, although knowledgeable, uses lingo that makes it hard for the receiver to understand what is being said. This particular characteristic can be most detrimental when communicating with community members. If the language is too high level, the audience most certainly will not be able to listen for understanding, defeating the whole purpose of engaging the community.

The Clincher

This speaker clinches onto the podium or microphone so tightly it appears they are hanging on for dear life. Like with the 'peacock' this behavior conveys nervousness to the receiver.

The Disorganized Artist

This speaker is disorganized with notes and ideas and appears to ramble. Speaking without purpose or a clear goal will confuse the listeners. Confusion is not a feeling you want to conjure in your audience, as they will begin to question the foundation of your expertise.

Group Facilitation

Prevention professionals are often called to lead prevention efforts, requiring us to facilitate meetings. A facilitator is someone who has been designated to preside over, manage, and navigate the meeting process. There are six roles of an effective facilitator (Hogan, 2003, pp. 244–245):

- **Encourage participation from all.** It is important to not let the talkers dominate the conversation and to encourage the quiet folks to share their ideas.
- **Foster effective listening.** Now that you are knowledgeable on the various ways a listener can be distracted, you want to create an environment that does not distract from the listening experience.
- **Clarify goals and agenda.** A well-conceived agenda prepares the group for the business at hand and assures an expedient and productive meeting.
- **Balance individual needs with group tasks.** Often our work brings together people from many different sectors of society. To that end, there may be times when a community partner's specific agenda is not in direct alignment with the work of the overarching group. For example, a

community partner may be passionate about prioritizing opioid overdose prevention due to a loss in their family. However, the local data shows marijuana use as the primary substance misuse problem in the community. The community partner might request the coalition shift their focus away from marijuana, to prioritize opioid overdose prevention.

- **Encourage shared leadership.** This role is vital to the sustainability of prevention efforts. Without shared leadership, our efforts cease when the leader leaves the project. 'It is not the job of the facilitator to take responsibility for every task generated by the group' (Hogan, 2003, p. 245).
- **Share the facilitator role with others.** This is connected to the previous role of encouraging shared leadership. Providing opportunities for share facilitation creates collective ownership. This ultimately improves the sustainability of our efforts.

Leadership Styles

Leadership is a process by which one person persuades others to accomplish specific tasks, and is often considered the most important characteristic of an effective leader. Without leadership, it would be nearly impossible to get anything done or overcome any obstacles that may come up in life. By this definition, the leaders do not DO everything. It is the members of the team that actually do the work, and the leader guides those efforts by holding the vision at the forefront of everyone's mind. So often, leaders do most of the work, creating an environment that ensures failure, primarily because the leader is overworked and burned out. Effective leadership is another critical skill in sustaining prevention efforts. Ideally, an effective leader can discern and use the best style appropriate for a particular situation, thus making the leader adaptive. Following are four categories of leaders, all having their unique strengths and limitations.

The Director

Typically, the leader makes decisions on their own, gives explicit instructions to others, follows up with close supervision, and values followers who comply with their wishes. This style is helpful when uniform results are desired. For example, this style works well when teaching new staff how to implement a curriculum. However, the weakness of this style is that this type of leader can appear dominating when people already know what to do or want more responsibility.

The Problem Solver

Involving group members in the problem-solving process, these leaders are good at listening to the issues and challenges and making decisions based on the recommendation(s) of the group. The leader makes the ultimate decision but involves others in the process. The limitation of this style is that the problem solver can get overwhelmed by all the details and over-involved in processes that are not necessary, which can be perceived by staff as a waste of time.

The Developer

The developer is a very good listener, is great at asking questions, and empowers staff to make their own decisions. Their style challenges staff to grow and learn how to solve their own problems. Competent employees will feel valued and motivated to solve problems on their own. The weakness of this style is that the leader can appear over accommodating by listening too much and letting others make decisions that should be made by the leader. Novice staff members looking for explicit detail on the functions of the job may not respond well to this style.

The Delegator

This leader designates meaningful responsibilities to others and entrusts them to handle assignments on their own. Decision-making occurs at the staff level, and the delegator simply guides the process. The weakness of this style is that when people feel overwhelmed, they are likely to accuse this type of leader of abdicating their responsibility to someone else.

Media and Prevention

Media has always played an integral role in our work. We have leveraged the media to build general awareness of problems and to create direct messages to encourage the individual to change perspectives and behavior regarding the use of alcohol, tobacco, and other drugs. Beyond increasing awareness, we use media advocacy to shift the focus from individual to collective behavior change by addressing community norms and policies.

In media advocacy, challenging conventional wisdom and public thinking is important. Mass media becomes the arena for contesting public policies and for shifting emphasis from individual behavior change to collective behavior change and policies. Media advocacy is a powerful tool for community change. As prevention professionals, it is our duty to assist reporters in sharing valuable information that can create shifts in how communities promote or discourage alcohol, tobacco, and other drug use. By using specific media-related skills, prevention professionals can provide the media with interesting information and stories that strategically support our prevention agenda. Let's discuss these skills in more detail.

Research

It is important for those using media advocacy to have current, relevant facts and figures on hand with the ability to clearly articulate and discuss their implications for alcohol, tobacco, and other drug issues. Reporters and editors are more likely to contact people they know who have access to reliable facts when they are researching a story. You want to be that resource for the reporters in your community.

In addition to gathering research on topics of specific interest, media advocates must also understand how local media outlets operate. Which reporters are most likely to cover health issues? What are the names of relevant news editors? Who should receive a news release? Do your own research on your local media outlets. Learning how the media prefers to receive information pays off big time. Your ability to navigate professionally and authentically builds credibility and trust and could prove to increase your level of immediate access to media coverage and resources.

Creative Use of Epidemiology and Other Statistical Data

The creative use of epidemiology and other statistical data is a powerful strategy. It involves translating the research, from often dry or bewildering facts and figures, into attention-grabbing news. News must have some immediate relevance. In other words, facts must not only be correct but they should also be presented in a way that brings the issue home to the receiver. As we discussed in Chapter 3, data is a topic that creates anxiety in many prevention professionals, yet data is one of your strongest assets for assisting the media in educating the public. You want the data you provide to tell a story that anyone can understand. Consider learning about data visualization, which is strategically using graphics to help nonprofessionals understand data.

Framing the Issue

Like the creative transformation of data, framing the issue, or influencing the terms of the debate, is a useful strategy. With any topic, both sides attempt to frame the issue to make their positions seem most reasonable. For example, when media advocates point out the predatory nature of the alcohol and tobacco industry in vulnerable populations (ie: excessive advertising), the alcoholic beverage industry attempts to frame its position in civic terms. The debate shifts from 'Should communities of color be targeted by the ATOD industry?' to 'Should this industry have their First Amendment rights protected?'

Framing the issue is everything! And the right story can paint a picture to support prevention or place the ATOD industry in a positive light. When we work with the media, we should be aware of how the issue is framed, so as to shed light on the complexity of how substance misuse egregiously impacts community health while countering the position of the ATOD industry.

Gaining Access to the Media

The last skill is focused on how we gain access to the media. This involves watching for opportunities to contact the media with timely information.

Contact may be established through a news release (with a follow-up tele-phone call), a letter to the editor, a guest editorial, or a telephone call to build interest in a story angle. Over time, media advocates can build credibility so that the media will contact them first when the possibility of an alcohol- or other drug-related story arises. With the advent of the social media world, gaining access to media outlets is getting easier. There are even indirect ways to stir media attention by using your own social media platforms and then 'tagging' media outlets into the communication piece.

Other Key Concepts

Media is such a broad topic. We engage with media all the time and so do the communities we serve. There are three additional concepts for us to explore in understanding the role of media in our prevention practice: Media literacy, social marketing, social norms marketing.

Media Literacy

Media literacy focuses on the skills and knowledge needed to analyze media messages critically and to become better-informed consumers. This is an extremely helpful skill for youth, as they are most susceptible to viewing media messages as 'real,' and oftentimes the media tends to glamorize unhealthy lifestyles. This can be easily seen by reviewing almost any alcohol or tobacco ad. These ads typically show people having fun with no consequences or regret. There are several examples of movies and TV shows that frame the negative consequences as epic adventures in which an often dangerous si-tuation is presented as satire or a funny story shared amongst friends.

Social Marketing

Social marketing is about the ability to 'sell' healthy behaviors. When devel-oping a social marketing campaign, prevention specialists need to consider the '4Ps' of marketing: product, price, place, and promotion (Walsh et al., 1993):

- **Product –** The product is essentially what you want the participant to 'buy.' In the case of substance misuse prevention, the product is the knowledge, attitudes, or behavior that the target audience should adopt.
- **Price –** The price is what the person must give up to receive the benefits. For example, the price may be the cost of separating oneself from peers that use substances. Or, the price of inconvenience a parent experiences when they adopt the habit of locking their medications or alcohol.
- **Place –** This represents the communication channel by which the target audience is reached (i.e., social media, radio, newspaper), and can also include the location of where the promotion is delivered, such as schools, churches, and community centers.

- **Promotion** – Promotion is the overall strategy or message used to persuade the target audience to pay the price for the product.

Traditional product marketing techniques include marketing analysis, planning, and control; these techniques include market research, product positioning and conception, pricing, physical distribution, advertising, and promotion. Here's an example of how the 4Ps of social marketing can be applied to a media campaign:

Product: Safely storing prescription medications

Price: The inconvenience of getting to medications that are locked up

Promotion: 'Locking up your meds is easy, convenient, and saves lives'

Place: Parent organizations, social media campaign, churches

Social Norms Marketing

Social Norms Marketing is used to promote and shed light on the healthy behavior practices of the majority. Media portrayals of substance use would have youth believing that 'everyone' drinks, smokes pot, or vapes. The perception is very far from reality. In fact, over the decades since prevention strategies began we have seen a decline in the number of youth reporting underage use (Levy et al., 2020). Check out the latest research (Figure 5.2) showing the upward trend of youth not using substances from 1976 to 2018 (Levy et al., 2020).

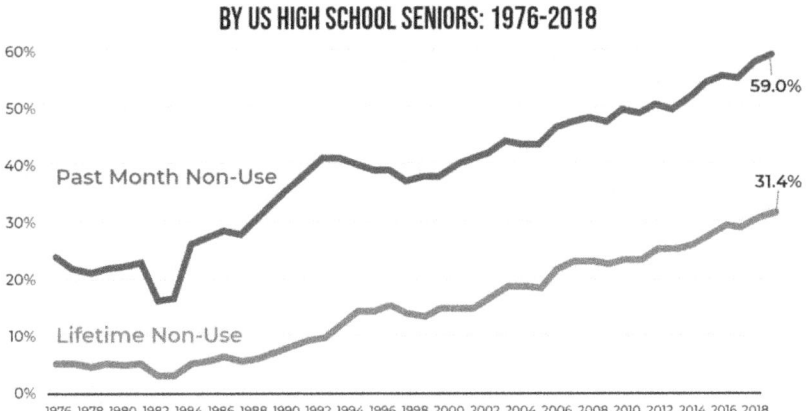

Figure 5.2 Trend of Youth Non-Use has inclined 31%–59%, 1976–2018.

Social norms marketing provides us an opportunity to address the perception that 'everyone' is engaging in unhealthy behavior. Using this strategy, we could create a campaign that might sound like this:

> Did you know that more than half of youth surveyed have NOT used any alcohol, cigarettes, marijuana or other illicit drugs in the past month? Most teens have sober fun! You're not alone!

Suggested Readings

Center for Substance Abuse Prevention (1993). Prevention primer: An encyclopedia of alcohol, tobacco, and other drug prevention terms. (DHHS Publication No. SMA 94-2060). Rockville, MD: National Clearinghouse for Alcohol and Drug Information.

Facilitating Meetings: A Guide for Community Planning Groups (2005). http://preventiontrainingservices.com/resources/Facilitating%20Meetings%20version_2005.pdf

Hogan, J., Gabrielsen, K., Luna, N., & Grothaus, D. (2003a). The media and prevention. In *Substance abuse prevention: The intersection of science and practice* (1st ed., pp. 170–209). Pearson.

Hogan, J., Gabrielsen, K., Luna, N., & Grothaus, D. (2003b). Communication strategies. In *Substance abuse prevention: The intersection of science and practice* (1st ed., pp. 233–251). Pearson.

References

Hogan, J.G. (2003). *Communication Strategies*. Boston: Pearson Educations, Inc.

IC&RC (2013, May 2). *IC&RC announces new prevention specialist job analysis*. Retrieved from IC&RC: https://internationalcredentialing.org/news/1374741

Levy, S., Campbell, M.D., Shea, C.L., DuPont, C.M., & DuPont, R.L. (2020). Trends in substance nonuse by high school seniors: 1975–2018.*Pediatrics, 146*(6). 10.1542/peds.2020-007187

Walsh, D.C., Rima, E.R., Moeykens, B.A., & Moloney, T.W. (Summer, 1993). Social marketing for public health. *Health Affairs*, 104–119.

6 Domain IV: Community Organization

Self-Assessment: Perceived Competency

Rate your knowledge/skill using the five-point scale (Table 6.1).

1 = Not at all knowledgeable/skilled, to 5 = Extremely knowledgeable/skilled

Table 6.1 Domain IV: Community Organization Accounts for 15% of the Test Questions

	1	2	3	4	5
Identify the community demographics and norms.	☐	☐	☐	☐	☐
Identify a diverse group of stakeholders to include in prevention programming activities.	☐	☐	☐	☐	☐
Build community ownership of prevention programs by collaborating with stakeholders when planning, implementing, and evaluating prevention activities.	☐	☐	☐	☐	☐
Offer guidance to stakeholders and community members in mobilizing for community change.	☐	☐	☐	☐	☐
Participate in creating and sustaining community-based coalitions.	☐	☐	☐	☐	☐
Develop or assist in developing content and materials for meetings and other related activities.	☐	☐	☐	☐	☐
Develop strategic alliances with other service providers within the community.	☐	☐	☐	☐	☐
Develop collaborative agreements with other service providers within the community.	☐	☐	☐	☐	☐
Participate in behavioral health planning and activities.	☐	☐	☐	☐	☐

Community involvement in prevention strategies ensures that the work is customized to meet the expressed, implicit needs of the community, while also embedding accountability and ownership of the community to address the problem, empowering the community to mobilize for action, implementing the identified solutions. In turn, community involvement creates the roots of a sustainable program, so the prevention work continues beyond the life cycle of a grant or a particular job position. This requires knowledge of community readiness, community mobilization, and coalition development. Involving the

DOI: 10.4324/9781003053941-8

broader community in prevention planning is critical and is, unfortunately, a forgotten element in the work we do. The best quote I've heard to truly describe the essence of this chapter is: 'Nothing about us, without us.' In the world of prevention work, community involvement is essential to success, as we are reminded by the well-known African proverb, 'It takes a village!' Community involvement includes everything from organizing and planning to enhance efficiency and effectiveness of service implementation – all of which help aid in fortifying interagency collaborations, synergistic coalition building, and forging competent, well-endowed networks. Listed are just some of the activities that can be done within the domain of community involvement! In this chapter, you will learn about:

- Community Readiness
- Effective Coalitions
- Coalition Development
- Coalition Management
- Building Consensus

Community Readiness

Community readiness was first mentioned in Chapter 3 in connection with Domain I. It is brought up again here because anytime you are doing community organizing, it is extremely important to assess the readiness of your community, as it will determine whether your community is even open to the work that you want to do. For example, if you are trying to get people involved with an initiative and they are still learning about certain concepts, then this may not be the best time for them to participate. That said, it is imperative to review the nine stages of community readiness in Chapter 3 as it is absolutely crucial for us as organizers and advocates to be familiar with these concepts before we move into coalition building. So often we start our work and give little consideration to the community's readiness to address a specific problem. This is a recipe for ineffective community engagement.

Effective Coalitions

What are the ingredients that make a coalition effective?

For this, I would like to reference the six elements of effective coalitions, a resource developed by the Prevention Technology Transfer Center, to better understand how to improve the performance of a coalition. Let's take a look at each of these in more depth (PTTC, 2019).

Goal Directedness

It is extremely important for coalitions to understand where you are going. This is how the group is made certain that all the activities engaged in are leading toward the desired outcomes. When the proper steps are completed in program planning, with clearly outlined goals, a comprehensive understanding of the strategies employed, and a clear vision and action plan for how to accomplish specific tasks and outcomes, the coalition is ready to mobilize the community for action. Goal-directedness assists the coalition in coming to a consensus on how to use resources. Remember, coalitions bring together diverse stakeholders, which means their interests are going to be different. Clear goals allow everyone to be on the same page about what you want to accomplish.

Cohesion

This concept is all about assuring that coalition members are on the same page, at both the community and organization levels. There has to be a feeling of unity and collective impact so that the different members of the coalition are working in harmony with each other. This is really how the magic happens in coalition work. If you have brought together the right group of committed, diverse stakeholders, and critical contributing community members, all working cohesively in collaboration, you will be able to accomplish amazing things.

Efficiency

Efficiency is such an important concept to think about. Our resources are already limited in the prevention space. In comparison, prevention receives the least amount of funding across the behavioral health continuum. We are a reactionary society that prioritizes *responding to* crisis versus *prevention of* crisis. This fact is evident in our continued struggle to keep prevention initiatives funded, but that is a topic for another book! Without improvements in prevention, we won't be able to slow down or eradicate the burden of addiction on our society. In the meantime, it is our duty to be efficient with the resources we are currently allocated. This is what allows us to do the greatest work and to be most effective. This means regularly reviewing your process data to find opportunities to improve your implementation strategies by removing what isn't working and paying attention to the indicators that show success.

Diverse Stakeholders

Coalitions remind me of an orchestra or a band, where you have multiple instruments that come together to create a beautiful harmony. This is what the element of diversity brings to our work. It brings talent. It brings new perspectives. It brings a community's lived experience, unleashing the power of community stories. It gives community members an opportunity to be recognized and valued for their contributions to solving problems, collectively. All of which are needed to tackle the many challenges that face us in our work. When we come together like this, anything is possible. The diversity of the stakeholders involved in our work significantly increases our available resources. Through strategic collaboration, we are able to leverage the resources of the collective to accomplish greater feats.

Opportunities for Participation

Remember, a coalition brings diverse people, businesses, and resources to the table. Despite this truth, so many coalition leaders carry the entire burden of leadership alone. It cannot be a situation where the coalition director does all the work because the membership will suffer. It is important that if you are in a leadership position of a coalition, that you've thought about the multiple opportunities for participation in accomplishing the work and recognizing the talents of the people at the table. This is so important. Oftentimes, coalition leaders forget to survey their membership for talent. Someone may be at the table representing a community organization, who is also talented in graphic design. They may be talented in strategic planning, evaluation, or marketing. Unless time is taken to truly evaluate the existing membership, the coalition (or community) may miss out on the hidden talents already in the room. It is important that people are not just at the table because of the job they have or because there's a Memorandum of Understanding (MOU) with their organization. Discovering membership talents will offer more opportunities for participation, engagement, and ownership of the coalition work.

New Skills

The great thing about coalition work is we are creating change in a community. It is always wonderful to provide an opportunity for obtaining new skills, acquiring enhanced learning, and personal and professional development because our field is based on science. Right? Our field is uniquely positioned and geared towards creating, inspiring, and initiating sustainable environmental change. There may be times when coalition members are coming to the table who have never done this work before or who only know the fear-based history of prevention. Our past is rooted in the narrative of scare tactics and judgments about morality and willpower. Many people only know prevention to be the D.A.R.E. (Drug Resistance and Education) program, the 'Just Say NO!' Campaign of Nancy Reagan, or the 'This is your brain on drugs' commercial from the 1980s. It is our charge to improve community and stakeholder knowledge of prevention science. Effective coalitions offer opportunities to learn new skills, obtain relevant training, receive technical assistance, and grow professionally.

Coalition Development

Forming an effective coalition requires skills that every competent prevention specialist should be able to accomplish. Here are seven steps to creating an effective community coalition (NHTSA, 2001):

1 **Search the landscape**
Just like we encourage communities to take a moment and review their current community assets, you must take the time to see what coalitions already exist in your community before deciding to form a new coalition. Save time and energy by collaborating with existing coalitions to accomplish a common goal.

2 **Brainstorm ideas on potential participants**
The composition of your coalition membership is extremely important to the success of your activities. You want to think about who should be involved in the work you wish to accomplish. Stakeholders are those individuals or organizations who will be involved in, affected by, interested in, or have power over an initiative in one way or another. Create a small group of thought leaders to assist you in identifying who should be recruited to be part of the coalition.

3 **Determine staffing, budget, and resources**
Very few things in this world are free, including the development, maintenance, and sustaining of a coalition. It is critical to the vitality of a coalition to have the financial resources to hire a coalition coordinator and cover any administrative costs connected with running the coalition (i.e., building space, equipment, technology, etc.)

4 **Invite people to join**
Coalition membership should encompass the stakeholders in the community and its members. It is important for leaders to constantly seek a broad representation of the community and continuously ask themselves: *'Who isn't at the table that should be?' Be sure that in your quest to involve diverse stakeholders, you don't 'tokenize' or bring people to the table just to meet your grant requirement. Be genuine in your invitation. Working with people requires a relationship. You can't skip that step, just because you have a grant that requires a certain audience to be 'at the table'.*

5 **Clarify expectations**
You want to have clearly identified what it means to join the coalition. Clear expectations of coalition membership allow a person to truly evaluate the degree to which they can be actively involved. Remember, this is not about having a lot of people at the table, it's about having the right people at the table.

6 **Develop a mission statement**
The moment you bring a group of people together, it is inevitable that there will be differences in opinions on the priority community substance problem. Developing a mission statement makes the direction and vision for the work of the coalition clear and accomplishable.

7 **Define goals and objectives**
Once the mission statement has been clarified, the coalition can develop the goals and objectives to ensure that mission is accomplished.

Coalition work can be challenging, and truly is the ultimate test of skills for a prevention professional. In that role, it is your responsibility to provide direction and guidance for the coalition without DOING all the work your-self. Remember our discussion on leadership in Chapter 5: *'Leadership is a process by which one person persuades others to accomplish specific tasks.'*

Coalition Management

Good leadership is promoting and balancing relationships among people and organizations. There are many tasks involved in providing good coalition management:

- Managing the internal process of the coalition
- Promoting openness and trust among members
- Helping meetings run smoothly
- Maintaining communication and connections among members between meetings

Facilitating Meetings

Running or chairing a meeting means more than just moving the group through the agenda. When you facilitate meetings, you are responsible for the well-being of the group and the members in it. That demands a certain amount of attention be paid to 'group dynamics' and other process issues.

Tips for facilitating effective meetings:

- When in-person, arrange seating in a circle or around a table so members can see each other. This creates a sense of belonging and collaboration, so that everyone is an active participant in the process. When virtual, create an expectation that everyone defaults to using their camera, except in situations where using a camera is not an option. This will help in making sure everyone is fully 'present' in the meeting.
- Start on time to respect those who showed up on time. This will naturally reinforce to the late-comers that this is a group that respects time. Be sure to consider how the meeting minutes (content) will be documented, as this will serve as a resource after the meeting for members to review the topics, duties, assignments, and action steps.
- Start with a welcome and introductions. Thank members for attending, and track attendance so that you have a record of who attended. Take additional time to welcome and introduce new members. There are times you may need your meeting attendance and/or minutes as proof to funders that your group is doing real work.
- Provide and review the agenda, while also offering an opportunity to make changes to the agenda before proceeding with the meeting. As the facilitator of the meeting, you should not be the only person talking or presenting the information. Your agenda should reflect that you are 'leading' the group, not doing all the work for the group.

- Establish ground rules so that everyone is on the same page about how to participate. Four powerful ground rules are: participate, get focused, maintain momentum, and reach closure. Consider placing this reminder on your agenda.
- Manage the discussion: This is where facilitation skills come in. Robert's Rules of Order may be a helpful resource to review. It is a format taught to assist with tools to run an orderly, productive, successful meeting.
- Identify future agenda items: keep track of new issues and action steps that will need to be addressed during future meetings.
- Evaluate the meeting: Leave about 5 minutes at the end of the meeting to evaluate the meeting. Use the feedback when planning future meetings. Make this an agenda item, so you are sure to create time for this important task.
- Close the meeting: Always end on time and on a positive note. Review actions and assignments, determine any new business, and set or remind members of the next meeting, logistics, and actionable items.

NOTE: With the social changes created by the COVID-19 pandemic, we will need to gain new skills in using virtual tools to facilitate meetings and engage community members. Our world has changed significantly as a result of the pandemic. There are many advantages and new possibilities when leveraging advances in technology to connect with folx virtually.

Building Consensus

The last element within management that we will discuss is building consensus. Consensus is a decision that everyone involved accepts as the best possible solution. That does not mean that everyone holds that decision as their own first choice, instead as partners agreed that it is the best choice. Consensus rather than majority rule promotes coalition effectiveness for several reasons:

- Commitment is increased because all partners stay involved, rather than withdrawing from the process in resentment.
- Knowledge is shared among partners.
- Sharing ideas and information broadens partners' perspectives.

Building consensus requires skill and patience. The skilled facilitator must keep the discussion going without rushing or taking control. Personal agendas and egos must not dominate to the point that not all partners are heard. The Facilitator must jump-start the meeting when it stalls and keep the focus on the issue at hand. Another key role of the facilitator is to organize data in a way that will help coalition partners reach a consensus on coalition goals and activities. This is a challenge even for the most skilled professionals. Develop a relationship with a seasoned professional to gain insight and get mentorship on these skills. Your leadership in community organizing will be of great value in improving community protective factors and reducing risk factors.

Suggested Readings

Capacity Primer: Building Membership, Structure and Leadership (2019). https://www.cadca.org/resources/capacity-primer-building-membership-structure-and-leadership

Handbook for Community Anti-Drug Coalitions (2019). https://www.cadca.org/resources/handbook-community-anti-drug-coalitions

References

NHTSA (2001). Community how to guide on…coalition building. Retrieved from https://one.nhtsa.gov/people/injury/alcohol/community%20guides%20html/Book1_CoalitionBldg.html#Community%20Guide

PTTC (2019, November 19). Six elements of effective coalitions. Northwest PTTC. https://pttcnetwork.org/centers/northwest-pttc/product/six-elements-effective-coalitions

7   Domain V: Public Policy and Environmental Change

Self-Assessment: Perceived Competency

Rate your knowledge/skill using the five-point scale (Table 7.1).

1 = Not at all knowledgeable/skilled, to 5 = Extremely knowledgeable/skilled

Table 7.1 Domain V: Public Policy and Environmental Change Accounts for 12% of Test Questions

	1	2	3	4	5
Provide resources, training, and consultation to promote environmental change.	☐	☐	☐	☐	☐
Participate in enforcement initiatives to affect environmental change.	☐	☐	☐	☐	☐
Participate in public policy development to affect environmental change.	☐	☐	☐	☐	☐
Use media strategies to support policy change efforts in the community.	☐	☐	☐	☐	☐
Collaborate with various community groups to develop and strengthen effective policies supporting prevention.	☐	☐	☐	☐	☐
Advocate to bring about policy and/or environmental change.	☐	☐	☐	☐	☐

Public policy and environmental change emphasizes the broader physical, social, cultural, and institutional forces that contribute to substance misuse problems and is one of the most powerful tools for prevention professionals in creating sustained community-level change. Implementing strategies from this domain have great potential for initiating change that could last for generations. In this chapter, we will review the following:

* Why do we use environmental strategies?
* The tools of environmental change.
* The use of media in support of environmental strategies.

DOI: 10.4324/9781003053941-9

Why We Do Use Environmental Strategies?

The prevention of substance misuse is a major public health priority. Environmental strategies offer well-accepted prevention approaches designed to change the context (environment) in which substance misuse occurs. Environmental strategies for preventing substance misuse involve changes to multiple levels of a community (i.e., schools, workplaces, recreational areas, etc.). Figure 7.1 shows the interconnectedness of community environment and health. So often our prevention strategies focus on the individual level with minimal consideration for the environment in which that individual lives, works, and plays. Take a moment to reflect on a thriving community environment. Think of the neighborhood, the schools, parks, grocery stores, and the physical built environment. Think of all the ways a person's health and well-being are nurtured by living in an environment with high protective factors. Now imagine the environment of those community members who are suffering from disparities and social inequalities. Can you see how different the environment looks for these two communities? If this is a foreign concept to you, just take a drive to the 'other' side of town and you will immediately see the difference. Much like the figure, you will see barren trees struggling to survive in unhealthy soil. Understanding this concept is paramount to understanding the role of the policy change and environmental strategies in creating sustainable change. When our efforts only focus on the leaves of the

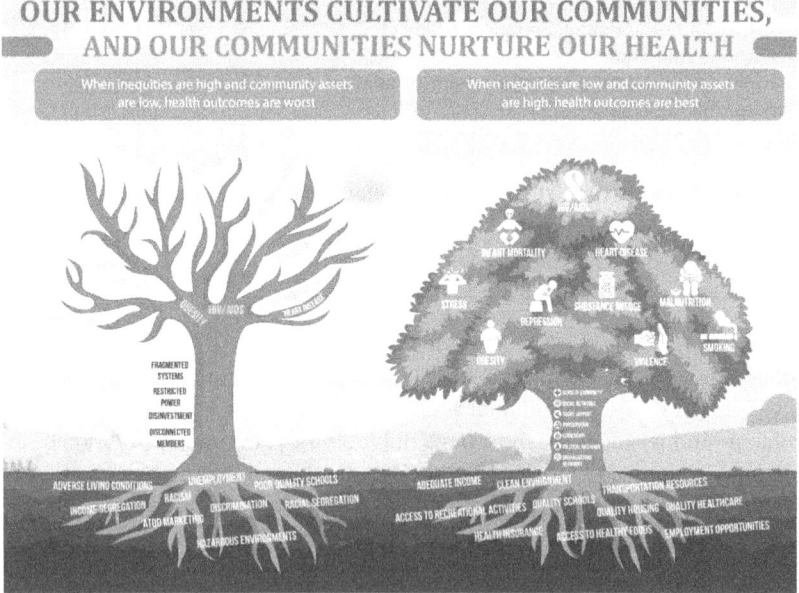

Figure 7.1 Correlation of Environments, Communities, and Health to Public Health Outcomes.

tree, we miss the opportunity to enrich the soil. Think about the prevention initiatives you're currently implementing. Are they focused on just the leaves of the tree? Consider what you could be doing to change the soil and roots of the community health problems.

So why are most of us continuing to focus on the individual level? There are three main reasons:

- Individual strategies are easier to count and track
- Most prevention funding supports individual strategies
- The history of prevention practice has focused mostly on the individual

The first two reasons are linked. Individually focused strategies allow you to track the numbers easily. You can make statements about how many people received services, collect satisfaction surveys from every participant in your program, and it is easy to show your program's reach. This ease of reporting and tracking is the main reason why prevention funding focuses primarily on supporting individual strategies. Individual strategies are based on the premise that substance misuse develops because of deficits in knowledge about negative consequences, inadequate resistance skills, poor decision-making abilities, and low academic achievement. The addiction field has a very long history of blaming the individual with language about 'will-power' or 'morality' as the cause for addiction. Prevention was born during a time when we didn't believe addiction was a disease. Addiction was thought of as one of the shortcomings of the individual and was shrouded in shame, secrecy, and stigma. Although we now have research to confirm that addiction is a disease and not a moral failing, this insight needs greater acceptance in the general population. It is our diligence as Prevention Specialists to check our own biases, ensure we are contributing to efforts that reduce stigma, and support the development of community initiatives that seek to shift the environment for lasting change. The greatest challenge in adopting this shift is to establish ways of tracking the changes created by environmental strategies. The reality is decreases in Adverse Childhood Experiences (ACEs), structural racism, unemployment, or other various inequalities take time. (Note: we'll come back to ACEs as an important concept connected to environmental strategies.) Much of our funding opportunities are short-term and count participation numbers instead of tracking environmental changes, which may not see results for years to come.

To make substantial changes in the environment, we must take a more holistic approach that recognizes and intervenes in all the interconnected facets of an individual's life and behaviors.

Environmental strategies for prevention are based on an understanding of environmental factors such as social norms, cultural values, physical settings, or policies that increase the risk for substance use and misuse. For example, if you have identified social access as the root cause of your community's underage drinking problem, then you could create strategies to shift the social norms and cultural values around providing alcohol to underage youth. In addition, consider what other factors are at play in the community (ACEs, social inequalities, etc.) that may, also, be contributing to the community's underage drinking problem. Environmental strategies have great potential for creating long-term impact and often require the collective input of multiple stakeholders to contribute to sustained community change. This is where knowledge and skills from Domain IV will be of great value in your work.

I want to take a moment to talk about Adverse Childhood Experiences (ACEs). Trauma, historical trauma, and Adverse Childhood Experiences are something that both research and practice in the field of substance misuse prevention, must begin to understand. That's because those who have experienced ACEs are more likely to experience problematic substance use as a result. Therefore, understanding how they can work together can bring about better results for all those involved. Although you won't be tested on ACEs, this is an important concept for improving prevention practice.

The term Adverse Childhood Experiences was created by Vincent Felitti, Director of the Department of Preventive Medicine at the University of California in 1995 (Davis, 2019). Felitti wanted to find out what caused weight gain and underwent studying 17,000 patients who went to a health care facility because they were obese. Although the research started by investigating obesity, it became immediately apparent the connection to a myriad of health outcomes.

The ACEs questionnaire has 10 questions and is separated into four types of experiences: emotional, physical, sexual abuse, and witnessing violence between parents or caregivers. The study shows a connection between an individual's exposure to these experiences early in life and negative outcomes, including mental health, substance misuse, violent behavior, crime, poor academic achievement, unemployment, or underemployment. It should be no surprise that the primary focus for the prevention of ACEs has been on the individual level. As mentioned earlier our field has a long history of focusing on the individual. ACEs have received some criticism for being individually focused, and thus we have seen and continue to see an expansion of the original idea. The best expansion of the ACEs concept was done by Positive & Adverse Childhood Experiences Connection (PACEs Connection), in which they propose 3 Realms of ACEs (Vein, 2019). Figure 7.2 shows the 3 realms and truly embraces the environmental approach.

The Tools of Environmental Change

Environmental change can happen in a variety of ways. Table 7.2 shows a side-by-side comparison of individual vs environmental strategies. Understanding the tools we use to create environmental changes can help us in implementing strategies that change the soil and roots of substance misuse problems.

Our best tool for change involves policy initiatives, which require understanding and using community organizing, mobilization, and advocacy tools. Environmental change has many benefits to communities: it creates jobs,

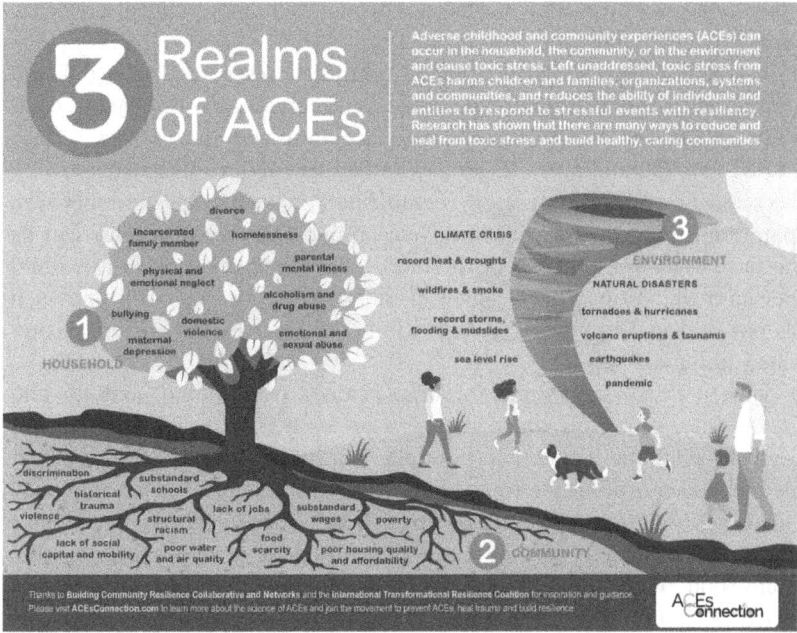

Figure 7.2 3 Realms of Adverse Childhood Experiences.

Table 7.2 Understanding the Difference Between Individual and Environmental Strategies

Individual Strategies	Environmental Strategies
Focus on behavior and behavior changes	Focus on policy and policy change
Focus on the relationship between the individual and alcohol/drug-related problems	Focus on the social, political, and economic content of alcohol/drug-related problems
Short-term focus on program development	Long-term focus on policy development
Individual generally does not participate in decision-making	People gain power by acting collectively
Individual as audience	Individual as advocate

improves public health, and provides better quality of life for all members of the community. Let's explore these three concepts and how they work together to create environmental change within a community.

Community Organizing

The concepts related to community organizing began in the previous chapter with the skills necessary for developing and managing coalitions. Community organizing is the process of empowering a community to take on an issue. To do this, organizers use tools including coalition-building, political advocacy campaigns, and public demonstrations.

First, coalitions are formed by bringing together representatives from different organizations in the community: businesses, civic organizations, religious communities, media, etc. For a comprehensive list of the diverse stakeholder, refer to the Drug-Free Communities 12-Sectors in the suggested readings section.

Second, the goal of community organizing is to create alliances between disparate groups to work collaboratively around shared goals. This can be done in many ways, but one of the most foundational skills is to listen and understand the various perspectives of different groups. You will find such skills outlined in Domain III, which will be of great use to you in accomplishing this goal.

Finally, it is also important for organizations with shared goals to find points of intersection on which they agree – even if this might not address everything everyone wants. For example, you might have several organizations mobilizing around the topic of youth development, however, they may all have very different views on how to accomplish that goal. Once you have community organizers at the table, you will then need to facilitate the consensus-building process. Building consensus will ensure everyone is working in concert to achieve a new vision for the community being served.

Community Mobilization

Community mobilization refers to any process by which communities mobilize their efforts to accomplish the agreed-upon goals. Whereas community organizing is like building a car, community mobilizing is like adding gas to that car. Without the gas, the car won't go anywhere, no matter how well constructed it is.

The benefits of community mobilization include strengthening the collective identity and solidarity of members, creating a sense of purpose, and increasing awareness about social problems among the people in the community.

Advocacy Tools

Advocacy is an underutilized tool for prevention professionals. Advocacy is the use of the political process to influence laws, regulations, and policies. When you think about what's needed to change the community environment, you can see the power of advocacy. However, due to fear of violating lobbying mandates, many providers do nothing and stay away from this strategy altogether. There is a rule preventing initiatives that receive federal funding from lobbying. Lobbying is a direct attempt to influence public officials and decision-makers. Lobbyists are paid professionals working for interest groups who support or oppose policies that affect the interests of the group they are representing. Typically lobbying involves asking policymakers to vote a particular way on upcoming initiatives. It's important to understand this difference to avoid lobbying activities and focus instead on advocacy. Advocacy is a less direct approach that can influence policies that support or oppose an issue. Advocacy may include creating petitions, writing letters, making phone calls, and going door-to-door in your community. It's important to realize the difference between lobbying and advocating because you can lose funding if there is any suspicion of crossing the line.

There are two types of policy change tools we can use when advocating: 'small P' and 'big P' changes. The small Ps are policy changes aimed at affecting the home, neighborhood and/or institution. These types of policy changes are often informal and don't focus on formally changing laws or ordinances. An example of 'small P' change would include an organization passing an internal healthy snack policy for all events. Another example might include a social service agency that requires all families to securely store medications, alcohol, or tobacco in the home.

The big P policies are aimed at changing public institutions and systems. These include formal changes to laws at the local, state, or federal level. Sometimes these policy initiatives can be used in conjunction with the small P initiatives. And oftentimes these types of changes require partnership with professional associations that have the freedom to lobby on behalf of the interests of the prevention field.

The Use of Media in Supporting Environmental Strategies

When it comes to environmental approaches, one of the best ways to communicate is through the media. We are living in a digital world, where many people get their news from social media, blogs, websites, TV, and even internet radio. It is important to be present in these spaces and be the voice providing accurate information, while also improving our reach to more of the community. It's no secret that reporters need content for their stories, whether they're covering politics or fashion trends. But what most people don't realize is how powerful an impact environmental approaches can have on society. Leveraging the reach of media to bring social awareness to our work is a strategy that deserves more attention than we have given it. Like with advocacy, this tool is rarely used because of 'stage fright' and the general concern of media misrepresenting the message of prevention.

Media plays an important role in the implementation of environmental approaches, and good relationships with media representatives and staff are vital to your long-term communication strategy. Traditional media outlets – newspapers, radio, and television stations – should continue as key partners with community coalitions. Advancements in technology now offer expansive channels for communicating and networking with your members, partners, and community at large. With so many journalists already looking for the next big story, you can capitalize on these reporters' needs and reach a whole new audience.

As mentioned in the Communication Domain (III), media can play a vital role in advocacy and social marketing. Pay attention to the way local media frame issues. Reports on drunk driving accidents involving teens often indicate that only the driver bears responsibility and rarely focuses on community issues such as the number of alcohol outlets willing to sell to minors, availability at community events, etc. Your message should move community members to support environmental strategies for sustained community change.

In order to build relationships, it is important to be proactive in the media world. If you're practicing the skills described in Domain IV, then the media should already be an engaged stakeholder in your prevention work. Create relationships with the media outlets and journalism schools in your community so you become their go-to resource for covering community stories connected to prevention strategies.

Suggested Readings

CADCA (2009a, September 1). Telling the coalition story: Comprehensive communication strategies | CADCA. https://www.cadca.org/resources/telling-coalition-story-comprehensive-communication-strategies

CADCA (2009b, September 1). The coalition impact: Environmental prevention strategies | CADCA. https://www.cadca.org/resources/coalition-impact-environmental-prevention-strategies

CADCA (2012, August 12). People power: Mobilizing communities for policy change | CADCA. https://www.cadca.org/resources/people-power-mobilizing-communities-policy-change

CADCA (2013, March 14). Strategizer 31 – Guidelines for advocacy: Changing policies and laws to create safer environments for youth | CADCA. https://www.cadca.org/resources/strategizer-31-guidelines-advocacy-changing-policies-and-laws-create-safer-environments

The White House (2021, September 23). Drug-free communities support program. https://www.whitehouse.gov/ondcp/dfc/

References

Davis, S. (2019, October 7). *A closer look at the adverse childhood experiences study (ACEs)*. Complex post-traumatic stress disorder foundation. https://cptsdfoundation.org/2019/10/07/adverse-childhood-experiences-aces/

Vein, M. (2019, December 5). *3 Realms of ACEs Handout*. PACEs connection resource center. https://www.pacesconnection.com/g/resource-center/blog/3-realms-of-aces-handout

8 Domain VI: Professional Growth and Responsibility

Self-Assessment: Perceived Competency

Rate your knowledge/skill using the five-point scale (Table 8.1).

1 = Not at all knowledgeable/skilled, to 5 = Extremely knowledgeable/skilled

Table 8.1 Domain VI: Professional Growth and Responsibility accounts for 15% of test questions

	1	2	3	4	5
Demonstrate knowledge of current prevention theory and practice.	☐	☐	☐	☐	☐
Adhere to all legal, professional, and ethical principles.	☐	☐	☐	☐	☐
Demonstrate cultural responsiveness as a prevention professional.	☐	☐	☐	☐	☐
Demonstrate self-care consistent with prevention messages.	☐	☐	☐	☐	☐
Recognize the importance of participation in professional associations locally, statewide, and nationally.	☐	☐	☐	☐	☐
Demonstrate responsible and ethical use of public and private funds.	☐	☐	☐	☐	☐
Advocate for health promotions and prevention across the life span.	☐	☐	☐	☐	☐
Advocate for healthy and safe communities.	☐	☐	☐	☐	☐
Demonstrate knowledge of current issues of addiction.	☐	☐	☐	☐	☐
Demonstrate knowledge of current issues of mental, emotional, and behavioral health.	☐	☐	☐	☐	☐

This domain focuses on understanding the foundational values of the prevention profession, which include maintaining the latest knowledge and expertise in prevention research and engaging in ethical practices. This chapter reviews the theoretical models used to develop prevention interventions, outlines the prevention specialist code of ethics, and discusses the importance of self-care in maintaining professional and personal balance.

DOI: 10.4324/9781003053941-10

Theoretical Models

The prevention field is 'predominantly informed by three theoretical perspectives: (1) risk and protective factor theory, (2) resiliency approach, and (3) developmental assets model' (Hogan, 2003, p. 14). In addition to describing these core theories, this section also provides an overview of some of the human development theories that also provide guidance for the implementation of parental strategies. Theories are valuable and should (Hogan, 2003, p. 14)

1 Identify the factors that predict substance misuse.
2 Explain the mechanisms through which the tenants operate.
3 Identify the internal and external variables that influence these mechanisms, including cultural factors.
4 Predict points to interrupt the course leading to substance misuse.
5 Specify the interventions to prevent the onset of substance misuse.

Risk and Protective Factors Theory

Risk and protective factors theory is a predictive theory, meaning it empirically states if certain conditions are present, a probable outcome may result. The idea is simple: identify the risks and create strategies to reduce the risk, while also identifying the protective factors and creating strategies to enhance those factors. There are four domains of focus for which prevention professionals can create such strategies: community, family, school, and individual/peer.

Let us think about the types of questions you might ask from each domain:

- **Community:** What is the neighborhood like? What are some of the most influential and effective community organizations in your area? Are they doing any work to reduce risk factors or create protective factors for youth and families living there?
- **Family:** How does parenting style affect children's outcomes? What level of parental engagement is needed to improve long-term outcomes? Are there viable, accessible parenting supports already present in the community?
- **School:** How do school policies and practices affect students' outcomes? How can we help to make schools more supportive for all students, including those who are at a higher risk of dropping out or being expelled?
- **Individual/Peer:** What is going on in a person's social environment that might put them at increased risk for developing certain problem behaviors? How do we improve resistance skills and boost confidence when we encounter negative peer pressure?

Prevention strategies based on Risk and Protective Factors theory are one of the most comprehensive courses of action and are necessary when aiming for sustained community change.

The Resiliency Approach

The resiliency approach is the study of how youth can thrive in adverse environments. Resiliency has been defined as a set of positive outcomes that have resulted from adversities and can even be seen as one's ability to cope with challenges or stressors. While many people believe that high-quality parenting is necessary for a child to develop resiliency, researchers have identified several factors that contribute to resilience (Hogan, 2003, p. 25):

- The age of the parent of the opposite sex (younger mothers for resilient boys, older fathers for resilient girls)
- The number of children in the family (four or fewer)
- Spacing between children (two years or more was best)
- The number and type of people available to help the mother rear the children (such as grandparents, aunts, or uncles)
- Steady employment for the mother, especially if she was a single mother
- The availability of a sibling as a caretaker in childhood
- The presence of a multigenerational network of friends, teachers, and relatives during adolescence
- Involvement in a faith community

Resilience is a complex process that involves both biological and social dimensions. The ability to bounce back from adversity by adjusting one's thinking, emotions, or behaviors ensures a better quality of life outcomes for youth with adversities in their lives. Understanding this concept can add great value to our prevention practices. You will often find the topic of resilience discussed as a solution to counter ACEs. Go back to the previous chapter to review ACEs and think about how the concept of resilience can assist us in creating initiatives that bolster community resilience.

The Developmental Assets Model

The Search Institute conducted a longitudinal study of over one million middle/high school students and developed a list of 40 assets necessary to create healthy, caring, principled, and productive young people. The study found that youth who possessed a high number of assets were more likely to thrive and less at risk of substance misuse, crime, violence, depression, or suicide.

These assets include the following:

1   Having at least one adult who is a role model (and being encouraged by that person)
2   Being able to discuss problems calmly with adults without fear of punishment or ridicule
3   Receiving social support from adults during stressful times

4   Learning how to resolve conflict nonviolently
5   Belonging to groups where they feel valued

These assets are divided into internal and external assets. Internal assets are the sense of belonging, hope, and optimism. External assets include caring adults, good education, financial stability, strong community bonds, and a well-maintained physical environment. The great thing about the Developmental Assets Model is that it has a self-assessment tool which can provide families with concrete ideas on how to improve their assets. Several studies have shown that when youth are more successful in achieving these 40 assets, they live healthier lives and enjoy higher levels of education success (Benson, 2003; Scales, 1999).

Human Development Theories

Prevention science is also molded by various Human Development Theories. It is important to have a working knowledge of the following theories and understand how their core concepts apply to prevention programming:

Abraham Maslow's Hierarchy of Needs

The concept of Maslow's Hierarchy of Needs is a theory that suggests that as humans' basic needs are met, they become more motivated to achieve higher levels of motivation. Also known as the *Hierarchy of Needs Theory*, this model was first proposed by American psychologist, Abraham Maslow, in his 1943 paper 'A Theory of Human Motivation' and further developed in his 1954 book 'Motivation and Personality.' According to the theory, human motivations can be classified into five categories or hierarchical level:

1   Safety – focus on survival, food, shelter, water, clothing, and the need for physical and psychological safety.
2   Belongingness and love – seeking connection, affiliation, and acceptance from others.
3   Respect and esteem – focus on developing competence, approval, and recognition.
4   Cognitive – developing a quest for knowledge, understanding, purpose, and an appreciation for goodness, justice, beauty, order, and symmetry.
5   Self-actualization – finding self-fulfillment and recognition of personal potential.

According to Maslow these five categories can be split into two types: the first being the **basic needs**, which must be met before someone can think about or have motivation for their **higher needs**, also known as **growth needs**. A person's basic needs include safety, feeling of belonging, respect, and esteem (the first three categories listed above). It is only after these needs are met that someone can begin to think about developing themselves on a higher level. It is through the development of one's growth needs that a person begins to discover their talents and unlock their potential. When adopting Maslow's conceptual model, prevention programs would need to adequately address basic needs as a precursor to helping communities develop their growth needs. This brings us back to the focus on *environmental strategies*. It is by changing the community environment that we are able to support individuals progressing to higher levels on Maslow's Hierarchy of Needs.

Erik Erikson's Psychosocial Development Stages

Erik Erikson's Psychosocial Development Stages are a set of eight stages that an individual will experience in their lifetime. Erikson believed that personality development is predetermined and occurs in the order of these eight stages, from infancy to adulthood. During each stage, there is a psychosocial crisis, which can either have positive or negative outcomes for the person's personality development, depending on how they react to it. Erikson saw this as an opportunity for parents to ensure their children grow up with the best possible chance at fulfilling their potential by guiding them through these critical developmental periods successfully.

Although you won't be extensively tested on the specific stages, it's good to know them and familiarize yourself with how this information applies to our work in prevention. Let's take a look at each stage.

Trust vs. Mistrust

The first stage begins at birth and lasts until your child is around 18 months old. Erikson believed this was the stage where we learn that other people are important in our lives and can be trusted. Erikson thought parents should encourage their children to explore but not give them too much independence to avoid becoming afraid or mistrustful of others.

Autonomy vs. Shame

The second stage begins at 18 months old and lasts until about age three. According to Erikson, children at this stage are focused on developing a greater sense of self-control. Erikson believed that parents should encourage children to explore new things but limit how much independence they have to prevent feeling like a failure.

Initiative vs. Guilt

In the third stage, Erikson asserted this stage begins around age three and lasts until about five years old. Erikson believed children during this time are focused on developing greater initiative skills as well as responsibility. In this stage, parents should encourage children to explore new things and take risks, but also limit how much independence they have so the child doesn't feel like a failure.

Industry vs. Inferiority

The fourth stage is thought to be between ages 5 and 12. Erikson believed children are focused on developing a greater sense of industry and skills. Erikson asserted that parents should help their children to explore new things, but not to the point where they feel inferior.

Identity vs. Role Confusion

Erikson stated the fifth stage is between the ages 12 and 18 years old. This is when Erikson said teenagers have true identity awareness and are making efforts to explore their independence. During this stage, parents should allow the child to have some sense of autonomy while at the same time guiding them through these difficult teenage years.

Intimacy vs. Isolation

This is the sixth stage and happens over an extended period of time, from ages 18 to about 35! Erikson said that people in this stage are focused on developing intimate relationships. Erikson suggested parents should support and encourage their children to explore intimacy as well as maintain a sense of individualism.

Generativity vs. Stagnation

The seventh stage takes place during middle adulthood between the ages of approximately 35 and 65. During this stage, people are focused on establishing and nurturing things and people, (i.e., children) that will outlive them. Erikson also stressed the importance of recognizing and appreciating what has been created so far in life, otherwise experiencing what is called a 'mid-life crisis.'

Creativity vs. Stagnation

The eighth and final stage takes place during the twilight years, when people are aged 65–80 and beyond! At this stage, people are reviewing the 'picture' of their life. Erikson stressed that we can appreciate our life as a whole and not just in parts. This stage also includes Erikson's theory on the 'creative old age.' Erikson maintained that people should continue to be creative during this phase of their lives- they need not fear overwhelming feelings such as loneliness or depression.

As you think of each stage, consider the population you most commonly serve. This information can help you better understand the developmental stage and modify your strategies accordingly. It's likely that many of your prevention interventions have been focused on the first five stages of Erikson's model. Remember prevention covers the life span, and understanding this particular human development model can assist us in creating prevention interventions for the stages of life past the age of 18.

Jean Piaget's Cognitive-Developmental Stages

Jean Piaget was a psychologist who studied how children learn and think. Jean Piaget's theory of cognitive development suggests that children move through four different stages of mental development. His theory focuses not only on understanding how children acquire knowledge but also on understanding the nature of intelligence. Jean Piaget believed that when children are in these stages, they think differently than adults would at the same stage of development. These developmental stages include the following:

1   Sensory-motor (birth to age 2): Stage one is characterized by infants' discovery of their own bodies and all aspects related to them – you could describe an infant as thinking through touch.
2   Preoperational (age 2–7): In stage two, children are capable of symbolic thought but cannot yet consolidate their thinking. This is thought of as a transitional phase where the learning of language is developed.
3   Concrete Operations (age 7–11): Piaget believed children in stage three are capable of symbolic or representational thought and can use logical operations, but they still cannot think abstractly. This is an important concept to remember when working with young audiences.
4   Formal Operations (age 11–15): In stage five, children can think abstractly – or that they understand the distinction between reality and fantasy. This is defined as the point when an individual's cognitive structures have reached maturity (Hogan, 2003, p. 150).

Additionally, Piaget coined several terms that help us understand how this process of cognitive development occurs:

Schema – describes the cognitive process of organizing information from the environment to make is easy to reference in the future. Schemata (plural for schema) are updated as the child ages and gains new knowledge.

Assimilation – the process of adding new information to an existing schema.

Accommodation – the process of change one's thinking when new information does fit into an existing schema.

Equilibrium – describes the cognitive balancing between assimilation and accommodation.

Disequilibrium – an imbalance between assimilation and accommodation.

Equilibration – describes the process of moving from disequilibrium to equilibrium.

Albert Bandura's Social Learning Theory

The Social Learning Theory of Albert Bandura emphasizes the importance of observing and modeling the behaviors, attitudes, and emotional reactions of others. Social Learning Theory explains human behavior in terms of continuous reciprocal interaction between cognitive, behavioral, and environmental influences. There are four stages of observational learning:

1   Attention
2   Retention
3   Motor Reproduction, and
4   Motivation

This theory supports initiatives designed for parents and caregivers to be positive role models, as the highest level of observational learning is achieved by first organizing and rehearsing the modeled behavior of the adults in a child's life. This theory also conceptualizes the idea that individuals are more likely to adopt a modeled behavior if it results in outcomes they value (ie: parental approval or disapproval). And finally, this theory also suggests that individuals are more likely to adopt a *modeled behavior* if the model is similar to the observer, has admired status, and the behavior has functional value. Programs such as Big Brothers Big Sisters were modeled after this theoretical framework.

Prevention Ethics

The Prevention Code of Ethics provides standards for how we should operate as professionals, and was originally developed by the former National Association of Prevention Professionals and Advocates. Later, revised and formalized by the Prevention Think Tank, and was officially adopted in 2011, by the International Certification & Reciprocity Consortium (IC&RC). The IC&RC are responsible for our credentialing exam. Our Prevention Code of Ethics was later revised in 2017, and the content in this chapter reflects the most updated ethical principles for prevention professionals.

Before we dive into the principles, let's first define two core terms for understanding how ethical principles are practiced: *Values and Principles*.

* **Values** are deeply held ideals and convictions that are influenced by culture and where you live. Every single one of us has our own set of values such as honesty, respect, hard work, loyalty, spirituality, or family first.

Values play an important role in ethics. You will always bring your own personal values to every situation, so it's important to have a clear inventory of your own values.

- ***Principles*** reflect the thoughts of an individual or group as to what behaviors are considered right or wrong conduct. Our principles are a set of guidelines that we all agree to as professionals.

There may be circumstances where you are in an ethical dilemma that conflicts with your values, and this is where nuanced situations occur. For example: Let's say you are currently getting near the end of a grant cycle, and there's a major report due. However, you're a parent, and your child gets sick. This situation may create a conflict for you, where if you hold the value of family first, before work, you will choose to leave the job in order to take care of your child and find alternative options for the job to get the work done. However, if you're someone who values work first, before family, you would stay at work to meet the deadline and find a sitter, family member, or someone you trust to deal with handling your child's illness. We are not drawing a conclusion that there is a right or wrong response in this particular situation, the point is to remind us that in our creating and abiding by ethical standards, there are times that making decisions professionally can be challenging when in conflict with our personal values.

Let us review the latest version of the Prevention Code of Ethics (2017), to gain a more in-depth understanding. In between each principle, I provide commentary to further explain the concept.

Preamble

The principles of ethics are models of exemplary professional behavior. These principles of the Prevention Think Tank Code express prevention professionals' recognition of responsibilities to the public, to service recipients, and to colleagues within and outside of the prevention field. They guide prevention professionals in the performance of their professional responsibilities and express the basic tenets of ethical and professional conduct. The principles call for honorable behavior, even at the sacrifice of personal advantage. These principles should not be regarded as limitations or restrictions, but as goals toward which prevention professionals should constantly strive. They are guided by core values and competencies that have emerged with the development of the prevention field.

Principle 1: Nondiscrimination

A prevention specialist shall not discriminate against service recipients or colleagues based on race, religion, national origin, sex, age, sexual orientation, gender identity, economic condition or physical, medical or mental disability. A prevention specialist should broaden his or her understanding and acceptance of cultural and individual differences, and in so doing render services and provide information sensitive to those differences.

Prevention specialists shall be knowledgeable about disabling conditions, demonstrate empathy and personal emotional comfort in interactions with participants with disabilities, and make available physical, sensory, and cognitive accommodations that allow individuals with disabilities to receive services. Prevention specialists should comply with all local, state, and Federal laws regarding the accommodation of individuals with disabilities.

Essentially, nondiscrimination means we are avoiding and preventing discrimination, making sure we comply with all anti-discrimination laws and regulations while embedding cultural competence in all that we do. Please refer back to Chapter 2 to garner a deeper dive into the term cultural competence. I would venture to say that a core component of being non-discriminatory is for every prevention professional to take an implicit bias test. Everyone has biases. It is an inherent part of being human. However, when these biases are based on race, ethnicity, gender, or other factors, they can have a negative impact on individuals and society as a whole. This is known as implicit bias. Implicit bias refers to the attitudes or beliefs that we hold subconsciously about certain groups of people. This can lead us to act in ways that are discriminatory, even if we are not aware of it. For example, studies have shown that people are more likely to associate Black men with violence than White men, even if they are shown identical pictures. This type of bias can affect everything from how children are treated in school to hiring decisions. The first step to tackling implicit bias is to become aware of it. We all have the ability to recognize and change our own biases. By increasing our understanding of these issues, we can make our world a fairer and more just place for everyone. Given our history of multiple types of discrimination (gender, sexuality, race, religion, economic status), we must create an explicit intention to rid ourselves of implicit bias so it doesn't get in the way of our work.

Principle 2: Competency

Prevention specialists shall master their prevention specialty's body of knowledge and skill competencies, strive continually to improve personal proficiency and quality of service delivery, and discharge professional responsibility to the best of their ability. Competence includes a synthesis of education and experience combined with an understanding of the cultures within which prevention application occurs. The maintenance of competence requires continual learning and professional improvement throughout one's career.

Incompetence includes but is not limited to a substantial lack of knowledge or ability to discharge professional obligations within the scope of the prevention profession or a substantial deviation from the standards of skill ordinarily possessed and applied by professional peers acting in the same or similar circumstances.

A   Professionals should be diligent in discharging responsibilities. Diligence imposes the responsibility to render services carefully and promptly, to be thorough, and to observe applicable technical and ethical standards.

B   Due care requires a professional to plan and supervise adequately and evaluate to the extent possible any professional activity.

C   A prevention specialist should recognize limitations and boundaries of competencies and not use techniques or offer services outside of their competencies. Each professional is responsible for assessing the adequacy of his or her own competence for the responsibility to be assumed. When asked to perform such services, a prevention specialist shall, to the best of their ability, refer to an appropriately qualified professional. When no such professional exists, a prevention specialist shall clearly notify the requesting person/organization of the gap in services available.

D   Ideally, prevention specialists should be supervised by competent senior prevention specialists. When this is not possible, prevention specialists should seek peer supervision or mentoring from other competent prevention specialists.

E   When a prevention specialist has knowledge of unethical conduct or practice on the part of an agency or prevention specialist, they have an ethical responsibility to report the conduct or practices to funding, regulatory, or other appropriate bodies.

F   A prevention specialist should recognize the effect of impairment on professional performance and should be willing to seek appropriate professional assistance for any form of substance misuse, psychological impairment, emotional distress, or any other physical-related adversity that interferes with their professional functioning.

The second principle, Competency, directs us to be diligent in discharging our responsibilities, thorough in our service provision, and regularly observe the standards that make us competent professionals. This is the situation where the word competence really holds value. Essentially, it means we are applying best practices in our work, engaging in ongoing professional development, and recognizing the scope and limitations of our own professional competence. This becomes extremely important to think about, primarily because in prevention, we will often work in tandem with folks in treatment, harm reduction, and recovery. In these coworking spaces, it can be very tempting to blur the lines. However, it is extremely important to remember that we are prevention specialists. We are not credentialed to provide any type of counseling or therapy. That is why amongst our strategies, we have problem identification and referral (refer to Chapter 3 to review the CSAP strategy). It's crucial to recognize the scope and limitations of our own professional competencies.

Two concepts I would like to highlight are in regards to accountability. First, *when we have knowledge of unethical conduct or practices of other prevention specialists, we have an ethical obligation to report that misconduct.* This is probably one of the most challenging things to do when it comes to being an ethical provider. Understandably, there is anxiety connected to to address the unethical conduct of colleagues. If you find yourself in such a predicament, I encourage you to do the right thing and have a conversation with your state board about your concern. And, lastly, *when we recognize the effect of impairment on professional performance and seek appropriate professional assistance*, this takes great courage If we notice impairments of any kind (psychological, social, mental, substance misuse) happening to ourselves, we must take initiative to recognize the need for seeking help and get appropriate treatment.

Principle 3: Integrity

To maintain and broaden public confidence, prevention specialists should perform all responsibilities with the highest sense of integrity. Personal gain and advantage should not subordinate service and the public trust. Integrity can accommodate the inadvertent error and the honest difference of opinion. It cannot accommodate deceit or subordination of principle.

A All information should be presented fairly and accurately. Each professional should document and assign credit to all contributing sources used in published material or public statements.

B Prevention specialists should not misrepresent either directly or by implication professional qualifications or affiliations.

C Where there is evidence of impairment in a colleague or a service recipient, a prevention specialist should be supportive of assistance or treatment.

D Prevention specialists should not be associated directly or indirectly with any service, products, individuals, and organizations in a way that is misleading.

E Prevention specialists should demonstrate integrity through dutiful cooperation in the ethics process of their certifying authority.

    1 Prevention specialists must cooperate with duly constituted professional ethics committees and promptly supply necessary information unless constrained by the demands of confidentiality.

    2 Grounds for discipline include failing to cooperate with an investigation by interfering with an investigation or disciplinary proceeding by willful misrepresentation of facts before the disciplining authority or its authorized representatives; by use of threats or harassment against any participant to prevent them from providing evidence in a disciplinary proceeding or any person to prevent or attempt to prevent a disciplinary proceeding or other legal action from being filed, prosecuted or completed; failing to cooperate with a board investigation in any material respect.

    3 Applicants for prevention certification are required to report any previous ethical violations from other disciplines or jurisdictions during the application process. The Ethics Committee is responsible

for making a recommendation concerning the application. The applicant is responsible for providing any additional information needed to make a determination on the application.

4   If a prevention specialist is cited for an ethical violation from another discipline or jurisdiction, they must immediately report the violation to their certifying authority.

5   As employees or members of organizations, prevention specialists shall refuse to participate in an employer's practices that are inconsistent with the ethical standards enumerated in this Code.

F   Prevention specialists shall not engage in conduct that does not meet the generally accepted standards of practice for the prevention profession including but not limited to, incompetence, negligence, or malpractice.

1   Falsifying, amending, or making incorrect essential entries or failing to make essential entries of services provided.

2   Acting in such a manner as to present a danger to public health or safety, or to any participant including, but not limited to, impaired behavior, incompetence, negligence, or malpractice, such as

   1   Failing to comply with a term, condition, or limitation on a certification or license.

   2   Suspension, revocation, probation, or other restrictions on any professional certification or licensure imposed by any state or jurisdiction, unless such action has been satisfied and/or reversed.

   3   Administering to oneself any controlled substance not prescribed by a doctor, or aiding and abetting another person in the use of any controlled substance not prescribed to that person.

   4   Using any drug or alcoholic beverage to the extent or in such manner as to be dangerous or injurious to self or others, or to the extent that such use impairs the ability of such person to safely provide professional services.

   5   Using drugs while providing professional services.

G   Prevention specialists make financial arrangements for services with service recipients and third-party payers that are reasonably understandable and conform to accepted professional practices. Prevention specialists:

1   Do not offer, give or receive commissions, rebates, or other forms of remuneration for the referral of program participants.

2   Do not charge excessive fees for services.

3   Disclose any fees to participants at the beginning of services.

4   Do not enter into personal financial arrangements with direct program recipients.

5   Represent facts truthfully to participants and funders.

6   Do not personally accept a private fee or any other gift or gratuity for professional work.

H   Prevention specialists uphold the law and have high morals in both professional and personal conduct. Grounds for discipline include, but are not limited to, conviction of any felony or misdemeanor during the period in which a prevention specialist holds a prevention certification, excluding minor traffic offenses, whether or not the case is pending an appeal.

Integrity really looks at how to maintain and broaden public confidence in us. When we are able to say that we are a field of integrity and we don't misrepresent our professional qualifications and affiliation, this gives the community greater confidence in who we are, our recommendations, and the services that we offer.

Be sure you are providing accurate information and giving credit where credit is due, in everything you do. It is also important to be sure you are being supportive to those who are needing assistance. There may come a time when you recognize that a colleague or a service participant has impairment issues. Part of integrity is recognizing those signs, providing support, and a referral to more services.

And finally, if you have a certification that expires, remove it from your email. You want to avoid any deception around your qualifications and affiliations. Make sure you're staying on top of any recertification process, and that any credential you have behind your name, and all information on your resume, is valid and accurate.

Principle 4: Nature of Services

Practices shall do no harm to service recipients. Services provided by prevention specialists shall be respectful and nonexploitive.

A   Services should be provided in a way that preserves the protective factors inherent in each culture and individual.
B   Prevention specialists should use formal and informal structures to receive and incorporate input from service recipients in the development, implementation, and evaluation of prevention services.
C   Where there is suspicion of abuse of children or vulnerable adults, the prevention specialist shall report the evidence to the appropriate agency and follow up to ensure that appropriate action has been taken.
D   Prevention specialists should adhere to the same principles of professionalism outlined in the Prevention Code of Ethics online as they would offline. With this in mind, the following are additional guidelines regarding the use of technology:

1   Prevention specialists are discouraged from interacting with current or past direct program participants on personal social networking sites. It is recommended that prevention specialists establish a professional social networking site for this purpose.

    a   Prevention specialists should not affiliate with their own direct program recipients on personal social media sites.

    b   Prevention specialists use professional and ethical judgment when including photos and/or comments online or in prevention materials.

    c   Prevention specialists should not provide their personal contact information to direct program recipients, i.e., home/personal cell phone number, personal email, social media accounts, etc. nor engage in communication with direct program participants through these mediums except in cases of agency/professional business

2   It is the responsibility of the prevention specialist to ensure, to the best of his or her ability, that professional networks used for sharing confidential information are secure and that only verified and registered users have access to the information.

3   Prevention specialists should be aware that any information they post on a social networking site may be disseminated (whether intended or not) to a larger audience, and that what they say may be taken out of context or remain publicly available online in perpetuity. When posting content online, they should always remember that they are representing the prevention field, their organization and their community, and so should always act professionally and take caution not to post information that is ambiguous or that could be misconstrued or taken out of context. It is recommended that employees not identify themselves as connected to their agency on their personal website.

4   Employees should be aware that employers may reserve the right to edit, modify, delete, or review Internet communications and that writers assume all risks related to the security, privacy, and confidentiality of their posts. When moderating any website, the prevention specialist should delete inaccurate information or other's posts that violate the privacy and confidentiality of participants or that are of an unprofessional nature.

5   Prevention specialists should refer, as appropriate, to an employer's social media or social networking policy for direction on the proper use of social media and social networking in relation to their employment.

E   Prevention Specialists must be aware of their influential position with respect to direct program recipients, and they avoid exploiting the trust and dependency of such persons. Prevention specialists, therefore, make every effort to avoid dual relationships with prevention participants that could impair professional judgment or increase the risk of exploitation. When a dual relationship cannot be avoided, Prevention Specialists take appropriate professional precautions to ensure judgment is not impaired and no exploitation occurs. Examples of such dual relationships include, but are not limited to, business or close personal relationships with direct prevention recipients and/or their family members.

1   Soliciting and/or engaging in sexual conduct with direct prevention participants are prohibited.

2   Prevention specialists should avoid any action or activity that would indicate a dual relationship and transgress the boundaries of a professional relationship (e.g., developing a friendship with a program participant, socializing with participants, accepting or requesting services from a participant, providing 'informal counseling' to a participant.)

3   Prevention specialists should not assume dual roles in a setting that could compromise the relationship with or confidentiality of participants (e.g., providing a skills group for students engaging in risky substance use behaviors, an 'indicated population,' and also teaching an academic subject where they are class members).

4   Prevention specialists avoid bringing personal issues into the professional relationship. Through an awareness of the impact of stereotyping and discrimination, the prevention specialist guards the individual rights and personal dignity of participants.

F   Prevention specialists should be aware of their influential position with respect to employees and supervisees, and they avoid exploiting the trust and dependency of such persons. Prevention specialists make every effort to avoid dual relationships that could impair professional judgment or increase the risk of exploitation. When a dual relationship cannot be avoided, prevention specialists take appropriate professional precautions to ensure judgment is not impaired and no exploitation occurs. Examples of such dual relationships include but are not limited to, business or close personal relationships with employees or supervisees.

1   Sexual conduct with employees or supervisees is prohibited.

2   Prevention specialists do not permit students, employees, or supervisees to perform or to hold themselves out as competent to perform professional services beyond their training, level of experience, and competence.

3   Prevention specialists who supervise others accept the obligation to facilitate further professional development of these individuals by providing accurate and current information, timely evaluations, and constructive consultation.

G   Prevention specialists make reasonable arrangements for the continuation of prevention services when transitioning to a new position or are no longer able to provide that service.

H   Prevention specialists should obtain written, informed consent from participants and/or parents/guardians for those under the age of 18 before photographing, videotaping, audio recording, or permitting third-party observations.

The Nature of Service principle is focused on how we interact with our service participants. Our primary rule is to make sure that we do no harm in our work and that we are supporting and strengthening protective factors. This is why the research conducted in the planning and assessment phases is so important. It ensures we are implementing services designed to *do no harm*. Remember, the work of prevention is community change. Thus, we should intentionally create opportunities for our service participants, communities, and the populations we serve, to be at the table when designing community change projects. That is what creates sustainability, produces community engagement, and strengthens community buy-in for the projects that you're working on.

The last concept to review in this principle is understanding what to do when you notice signs of abuse. It is very likely, that in the span of your career you will encounter a situation that calls for you to report abuse. It's important to recognize the part of our Code of Ethics that requires that any time we notice or have a suspicion of abuse of children or vulnerable adults, we report this evidence to the appropriate agencies. More details on reporting are covered under the next principle: *Confidentiality*.

Principle 5: Confidentiality

Confidential information acquired during service delivery shall be safeguarded from disclosure, including – but not limited to – verbal disclosure, unsecured maintenance of records, or recording of an activity or presentation without appropriate releases. Prevention specialists are responsible for knowing the confidentiality regulations relevant to their prevention specialty.

Prevention specialists make appropriate provisions for the maintenance of confidentiality and the ultimate disposition of confidential records. Prevention specialists ensure that data obtained including program evaluation data and any form of electronic communication are secured by the available security methodology. Data shall be limited to information that is necessary to and appropriate to the services being provided and be accessible only to appropriate personnel. Data presented publicly shall be distributed only in ways that protect the confidentiality of individual participants.

In prevention, we have confidential information, and it is our duty to protect and properly store that information. Confidential information can only be shared with proper permission from the program participant. As prevention professionals, it is our responsibility to know and adhere to confidentiality regulations. Confidential information acquired during service delivery should be safeguarded from disclosure, including but not limited to: verbal disclosure, unsecured maintenance of records, or recording of any activity or presentation without appropriate releases.

Let's review confidentiality regulation 42 CFR Part Two, which really focuses on confidentiality in two categories. *Any information about an individual's substance use* and *any information that identifies an individual as a participant in a program for substance users* are both considered confidential information. We cannot disclose directly or indirectly any type of confidential information.

Now, there are times and spaces when information can be shared without a release and it's always good to know when that is the case. Following are four examples:

- **Internal program communication.** For instance, let's say you're talking to your supervisor to receive guidance on a particular program. You can share information in that context.
- **Court order and criminal investigation.** In those particular instances, information is going to be released, however, you will have completed all the proper paperwork for the release of information to not be in violation of any laws. Sometimes there are situations of child abuse and neglect, which require mandatory reporting. Often, in these instances, you will not have a release and should contact your supervision immediately to discuss your concerns and start the reporting process.
- **Crimes involving a program.** Let's say, during a prevention specialist program you have a participant who commits a crime. Obviously, in that context, you can break confidentiality in order to contact law enforcement to get the help you need. The same thing happens in health emergencies. You can share necessary information with a medical professional in order to get an immediate emergency response initiated.
- **Research evaluations and audits.** No release is needed for these activities because it is a *time-limited situation* in which qualified individuals are accessing the data for purposes of an audit or program evaluation.

Principle 6: Ethical Obligations for Community and Society

According to their consciences, prevention specialists should be proactive on public policy and legislative issues. The public welfare and the individual's right to services and personal wellness should guide the efforts of prevention specialists to educate the general public and policymakers. Prevention specialists should adopt a personal and professional stance that promotes health.

Prevention Specialists should be aware of their local and national regulations regarding lobbying and advocacy and act within the laws and funding guidelines.

This last ethical principle is a very important concept in our ethical code. So often, the topic of ethics is focused on what to do, how to act, how not to act, and it's very internal and technical. This particular component really has to do with what we are doing as professionals to further our field, advocate for public policy, and be involved in legislative issues. This is the area, in which I would say, we can always use more work.

The main thing to consider is understanding that advocacy means taking action to support an idea or a cause and that as prevention professionals we are called to be advocates. Through our advocacy, we're educating community members, the media, and elected officials in order to raise awareness and increase understanding of key issues. This is what helps us mobilize support with the goal of creating positive change.

Often, folks are nervous about getting into the political space. We can be very active in politics, however, avoid lobbying. I want to explain and describe the difference between advocacy and lobbying. Advocacy is focused on educating and raising awareness. Lobbying is when you are making an attempt to direct a voting action in a particular way. The moment you begin talking about particular bill numbers or voting yes or no, you have shifted into lobbying.

As a side note, take some time to research what professional advocacy associations exist that you can join and become an active member! It gets you intermingled and engaged amongst other professionals and helps you better understand the value of advocacy. These are the six principles that govern our ethical standards and I encourage you to check out the full Code of Prevention, Code of Ethics, listed under the suggested readings.

Personal Wellness

Wellness and self-care affect the quality of work we provide. If you are unwell, you will not be able to give your best in your work, whether that be with coworkers or with program participants. SAMHSA's presentation of the eight dimensions of wellness gives a comprehensive look at the various aspects of wellness. Let's review each dimension:

1 **Social**

This dimension focuses on how we develop a sense of connection, belonging, and a well-developed support system. Social well-being is how we interact with other people in the community. It helps us form connections through friendships and family, gives us a sense of belonging, and allows for satisfaction in life. This dimension was significantly affected by the COVID-19 pandemic as we needed to practice physical distancing as a means of protecting our health. We are social creatures, and thus the connection is such an important part of developing a sense of community. What are some of the ways you have adapted your social life during COVID-19? Also, consider how your workplace social life changed? Think of what you are doing to regain and maintain healthy social connections. Building a healthy social dimension might involve asking someone out for lunch, joining an organization or club that you're interested in, and using assertive communication skills instead of passive-aggressive ones, which can lead to increased conflict between parties involved.

2 **Emotional**

Emotional wellness allows us to effectively cope with life and create satisfying relationships. Acceptance of one's feelings and coping with and expressing emotions in a healthy and adaptive manner is an important part of emotional wellness. Think of who you connect with for emotional support, or what do you do to relieve stress? People who have healthy emotions feel confident, in control of their feelings or behaviors, and are able to handle any challenges that may come up. The ability to navigate life challenges is the essence of resilience. Facing and working through tough situations builds resiliency, which helps us learn more about our strengths.

3   **Physical**

When the word 'wellness' is mentioned, physical wellness is probably the dimension that people think of most. Physical wellness is not just about being fit and healthy, but also includes the need for good nutrition and a safe environment. It is an essential part of health that includes eating nutritious foods, exercising regularly, managing weight, avoiding risky behaviors such as alcohol misuse or smoking, and, as much as feasible, avoiding environmental hazards from pollution to sunburns.

4   **Occupational**

Occupational wellness focuses on your personal satisfaction and enrich-ment received from one's work. This includes preparing and making use of your gifts, skills, and talents in order to gain purpose, happiness, and enrichment in your life. Look for opportunities to grow professionally and to be fulfilled in your 'job,' whatever that may be. As you think of your future and your occupational wellness you want to:

- Create a vision for your career goals
- Visit a career planning/placement office and use the available resources
- Talk to a mentor about career options

5   **Environmental**

Your environment can have a big impact on your health. The natural settings, social surroundings and things you come into contact with daily all contribute to how we feel in general. If the space where you spend most of your time feels cluttered or unorganized, it can be hard to concentrate and even inhibit your creativity. Enjoying good health includes occupying a pleasant, stimulating environment that supports well-being. This dimension also includes living in harmony with nature by understanding the impact of your actions on nature. As the planet braces itself for climate change, it is important that we take steps now in order to have a sustainable lifestyle. One way you can do this is by maintaining environmental wellness within your community and home- For example, recycling reduces wastefulness (community), while gar-dening provides fresh produce (home). Whether these aspects are present already, there's always room for improvement! Be sure to start small – think about what changes would make an immediate difference.

6   **Financial**

Financial wellness involves the process of learning how to successfully manage financial expenses. Learning how to maximize your financial wellness now will help you feel prepared to handle potentially stressful financial situations in the future. Financial wellness may be a dimension to which you are surprised is a part of wellness. Yet the lack of financial wellness can create all sorts of stress in a person's life and can create an imbalance in all the other areas of wellness. Keeping up with financial responsibilities can quickly become overwhelming, yet ignoring them will only increase feelings of stress and anxiety. Developing financially smart habits early in life is a valuable investment to achieve your future goals. I've often wondered why we don't see more prevention interventions that include partnerships with financial literacy programs, given how much of life perpetuate by need for money as a way to access resources.

7   **Intellectual**

Some of you may remember the famous slogan from the 1970s and 1980s: '*The mind is a terrible thing to waste, but a wonderful thing to invest in*' (Demby, 2013). Intellectual wellness is when you recognize your unique talents to be creative and seek out ways that will help stimulate and cultivate mental growth. Intellectual strengths allow us the ability, through engaging in various activities such as reading books or taking classes on topics of interest, to come up with new ideas for ourselves. Engaging in creative, stimulating mental activities, striving for personal growth, and a willingness to seek out and use new information, are critical activities to developing intellectual wellness.

8   **Spiritual**

The search for the meaning of and purpose of our life is natural. This creates our guiding beliefs, principles, or values that help give direction to one's life. Finding a spiritual practice includes

* Exploring/contemplating your spiritual side
* Allowing yourself and those around you the freedom to be who you/ they are
* Worshiping, prayer, meditation, etc.

Spiritual wellness is not just about your spiritual beliefs. It's also related to how you live every day and what matters most to you in life. A healthy spirit comes from having clear values that are important enough to pursue with self-confidence, while simultaneously feeling at peace internally.

Be sure to take time for your own personla self-care. The work of a prevention professional can be taxing, and some of use carry our own ACEs. As you focus on keeping yourself well, you are better able to help the communities you serve.

Suggested Reading

Hogan, J., Gabrielsen, K., Luna, N., & Grothaus, D. (2003a). Prevention research. In *Substance abuse prevention: The intersection of science and practice* (1st ed., pp. 14–41). Pearson.

Hogan, J., Gabrielsen, K., Luna, N., & Grothaus, D. (2003b). Incorporating human development theory into prevention. In *Substance abuse prevention: The intersection of science and practice* (1st ed., pp. 121–169). Pearson.

Hogan, J., Gabrielsen, K., Luna, N., & Grothaus, D. (2003c). Substance abuse prevention: The intersection of science and practice. In *The cultural context and ethics of prevention* (1st ed., pp. 103–120). Pearson.

IC&RC – PS (2021). Prevention Specialist (PS). https://www.internationalcredentialing.org/creds/ps

SAMHSA (2016). *Creating a healthier life: Step-by-step guide to wellness*. SAMHSA Store. https://store.samhsa.gov/sites/default/files/d7/priv/sma16-4958.pdf

References

Benson, Peter L. (2003). Developmental Assets and Asset-Building Community: Conceptual and Empirical Foundations, Developmental Assets and Asset-Building Communities (pp. 19–43). 10.1007/978-1-4615-0091-9_2

Demby, G. (2013, June 14). *New ads still warn a mind is a terrible thing to waste*. NPR. https://choice.npr.org/index.html?origin=https://www.npr.org/sections/codeswitch/2013/06/14/191796469/a-mind-is-a-terrible-thing-to

Scales, P.C. (1999). Reducing risks and building developmental assets: Essential actions for promoting adolescent health. 63(3) *Journal of School Health*, 113–110.

Part III

Practice Tests and Other Resources

9 Preparing to Become Credentialed

The decision to become certified is one we should all make! Certification adds a level of professionalism to our field that is important to improving the quality of our work, while also giving us the opportunity to advocate for consistent standards across the field. This chapter will provide information on the standard requirements to become certified as defined by the International Credentialing & Reciprocity Consortium. This chapter has two practice tests to assist you in checking your knowledge.

IC&RC Standards

Definition: IC&RC member boards define prevention as *a proactive process that empowers individuals and systems to meet the challenges of life events and transitions by creating and reinforcing healthy behavior and lifestyles and by reducing risks contributing to alcohol, tobacco, and other drug misuse and other related issues.*

Experience: Verification of one (1) year (2,000 hours) alcohol, tobacco, other drugs (ATOD) prevention-related experience.

Training: Verification of 120 contact hours of prevention-specific training. Twenty-four (24) hours of this training must be specific ATOD training. Six (6) clock hours of training in prevention-specific ethics is also required. Must have verification that hours cross all six (6) performance domains.

Examination: Passing the three-hour IC&RC prevention examination. The exam has a total of 150 questions; 25 are pretest questions and not scored. This is the weighted distribution of content across the six domains:

Planning and Evaluation: Domain I	30%
Prevention Education and Service Delivery: Domain II	15%
Communication: Domain III	13%
Community Organization: Domain IV	15%
Public Policy Environmental Change: Domain V	12%
Professional Growth and Responsibility: Domain VI	15%

DOI: 10.4324/9781003053941-12

Recertification: Includes the review of forty (40) continuing education hours for the purpose of maintaining certification. This process usually occurs every two to three years.

Please note: You will need to check with your specific state board, as states are allowed to make their own regulations on the credentialing process. For example, some states require credentialing and expect the process to be completed within a specific timeframe of entering the workforce. The Prevention Technology Transfer Center has a digital map providing more details on the requirements for each state: https://pttcnetwork.org/centers/prevention-specialist-certification/prevention-specialist-certification-states

Tips for Studying

Studying for a certification exam can feel like a daunting task. Here are some strategies I found most helpful:

- **Form a study group** – Have you ever heard the saying 'two brains are better than one?' I found this perspective extremely helpful in studying for this certification exam. Connect with other prevention professionals who are not yet certified.
- **Identify a mentor** – Having access to someone with more knowledge and experience than yourself will prove beneficial when you need clarification on specific concepts. You will be able to tap into their history of lessons learned.
- **Time your first attempt** – People always seem to worry they won't have enough time to finish the test. I find it helpful to set a timer when taking the test. This will give you a sense of your pace. Time yourself the first time you take the test and make a note of how it took you to answer the questions. Remember you will have 3 hours to answer 150 questions. The test of computer-based, allowing you to skip questions you don't immediately know. It is recommended to move forward and come back to questions that require more thinking.
- **Dissect each test question** – This certification exam is about the application of prevention knowledge. Sure, some of the questions are straightforward and simply ask you to identify the definition of a concept. However, I found a lot of the questions required me to understand multiple concepts to help me choose the best answer. Use your study group and mentor to discuss WHY an answer is correct or incorrect.
- **Leverage your learning style** – Learning is a complex process and it's unique for every person. Take some time to think about what you need to learn best. Discover your style and then start studying in a way that maximizes your learning.
- **Critically evaluate what you do on the job** – The concept of the examination should be reflective of what you're doing on the job. You

should be able to think about the work you do now and what prevention theory you're using to guide your professional practice.

- **Consider your need for special accommodations** – IC&RC provides accommodation for those needing modifications in how the test is administered. Be sure to reach out to your local board to make arrangements.

Practice Questions, Set 1

Two sets of questions are here for your review. These sample questions are reprinted from the '*Studying for Success: Preparing for and Passing the IC&RC Prevention Specialist Exam*' (EMT Associates, Inc., 2012). To ensure maximum understanding, an explanation for the correct answer is provided in the next chapter.

1   A needs assessment that uses information collected from interviews, focus groups, and/or observations involving document reviews to produce a descriptive report is called

   A   Qualitative data.
   B   Outcome data.
   C   Quantitative data.
   D   Indicator data.

2   One of the goals of prevention is to learn about the long-term effects on our culture. The type of assessment needed to measure these effects is called

   A   Outcome assessment.
   B   Cultural diversity assessment.
   C   Process assessment.
   D   Long-term assessment.

3   Theories of causation help to identify why youth begin using drugs. Substance misuse prevention program designers must determine what factors are involved. At the most basic level, these factors are

   A   Schools and communities.
   B   Family and peers.
   C   Individuals and family.
   D   Risk and protective.

4   It is important to match risk and protective factors in substance misuse prevention programming. Which of the following statements have a good match between risk and protective factors and programming?

   I   *A school-based program working on self-esteem with children who live in abusive families.*
   II   *A school-based program working on life skills with low-risk students.*

III *A school-based support group program for students who have violated school substance policies.*

    A   **I** only.
    B   **III** only.
    C   **I** and **II** only.
    D   **II** and **III** only.

5 Media campaigns dealing with prevention techniques affect audiences by

    A   Educating the public.
    B   Increasing problem awareness.
    C   Changing attitudes toward the behavior.
    D   Changing the behavior.

6 Targeted programs are

    A   High-impact, highly focused programs for risk reduction.
    B   Low-impact, broadly publicized programs for interdiction.
    C   High-impact, broadly publicized programs for intervention.
    D   Programs funded for a short time to serve a specific group.

7 The best description of the 40 Developmental Assets Model is

    A   Helps prevent risky behaviors in youth.
    B   Developed by the Search Institute and focuses on the strengths needed for success.
    C   Is based on resiliency only.
    D   Looks at the strengths of each person.

8 A thorough prevention needs assessment process should involve

    I   *Key stakeholders.*
    II   *Collection of consumption/consequence data.*
    III *Funding options.*
    IV   *Identification of target (affected) populations.*

    A   I only.
    B   III only.
    C   I and IV only.
    D   I, II, and IV only.

9 The Strategic Prevention Framework is used to

    I   *Prepare a needs assessment.*
    II   *Identify community resources.*
    III *Build capacity.*
    IV   *Select and implement an appropriate prevention approach.*

    A   **I** only.
    B   **I** and **II** only.

C **III** and **IV** only.
D **I**, **II**, **III**, and **IV**.

10 The IOM health care model defines three types of prevention approaches/target populations. The terminology that BEST reflects one of these types is

A Universal.
B Children of Substance Abusing Parents (COSAP).
C High-Risk Youth.
D Substance Users.

11 An example of an indicated prevention strategy includes

A Student Assistance Program (SAP).
B Media Campaign.
C Schools Assemblies.
D Social Norm Program.

12 The most important feature in creating a logic model is

A They try out multiple strategies.
B They enhance community involvement.
C They help you determine appropriate staffing patterns.
D They connect your outcomes and your goals.

13 The prevention planning structure using a five-step process that includes assessment, capacity, planning, implementation, and evaluation is known as

A Problem Identification and Referral Model.
B Social Development Strategy Model.
C Strategic Prevention Framework.
D Public Health Model.

14 Mobilizing community members to participate in a community prevention effort is an example of

A Community readiness.
B Problem prioritization.
C Coalition building.
D Community needs assessment.

15 You are planning to use a proven, evidence-based program, but realize it is not feasible to implement all of the program components. You should

A Not proceed at all with your choice.
B Consult with the developers to determine potential impact.
C Go ahead, as most programs can be modified to meet local circumstances.
D Add additional alternatives to fill out the missing components.

16   A prevention program that has been designated as a best practice means

  A   It has been adapted by many prevention programs throughout the country.
  B   It reflects the specific cultural needs of the community.
  C   It needs to involve a skilled, experienced program director.
  D   It has been shown through research and evaluation to be effective.

17   What is the best way to engage community members?

  A   Ask them for their advice.
  B   Get them involved in the planning process.
  C   Survey them.
  D   Conduct a focus group.

18   What level of networking and collaboration best describes the following situation?

  At a meeting, various after-school programs share their summer schedule with each other.

  A   Coordination.
  B   Communication/Networking.
  C   Cooperation.
  D   Collaboration.

19   If your community coalition lacks participation from a specific cultural group you should

  A   Go with the group that has volunteered to serve in your coalition.
  B   Invite them to your next planning meeting.
  C   Wait until the current coalition is completed with its work.
  D   Have collation members go to their community and ask them to participate.

20   In selecting a prevention program, what should you do?

  A   Select the program with community input.
  B   Base decision on what other prevention programs are doing.
  C   Base selection on the prevention literature.
  D   Select a universal-based approach.

21   A community is in denial when it

  A   Does not recognize it has a substance problem.
  B   Has no active leaders interested in the problem.
  C   Has not engaged in the collection and analysis of substance data.
  D   All of the above.

22   One of the most effective strategies to use involves scare tactics, presenting the realities associated with substance use.

  A   True.
  B   False.

23 A prevention strategy aimed at informing broad segments of society is called a

  A   Universal program.
  B   Selected program.
  C   Indicated program.
  D   Risk and protective approach.

24 A program that has been researched and found to be effective is known as

  A   Proven.
  B   Best practice.
  C   Promising.
  D   Excellent.

25 Ways you might encourage community readiness to address their local substance problem include

  A   Provide educational outreach to community leaders.
  B   Provide prevalence rates on substance problems.
  C   Conduct in-service training.
  D   All of the above.

26 A goal statement

  A   Specifies what and when something is to be accomplished.
  B   Is general and inclusive.
  C   Identifies who will do what tasks.
  D   Is the same as a mission statement.

27 An objective statement

  A   Is time-specific and measurable.
  B   Identifies specific individuals and their responsibilities.
  C   Is general and inclusive.
  D   Compares planned to achieved tasks.

28 A community readiness process

  A   Identifies community resources available for prevention activities.
  B   Summarizes substance use and problems associated with their use.
  C   Determines whether community members believe they have a substance problem or not.
  D   All of the above.

29 Consumption data is generally derived from

  A   Surveys.
  B   Archival data repositories.
  C   Prevention program records.
  D   Focus groups.

30 A gap analysis refers to

A   The difference of consumption patterns between adolescent youths from different age groupings.
B   The differences in available community resources as compared to the extent of the substance problems.
C   The number of current prevention programs as compared to the number of services available in prior years.
D   The difference in funding allocations for current prevention efforts as compared to the funding amount one year ago.

31 The greatest optimism in the development of substance misuse prevention activities has come from

A   Individualized prevention efforts.
B   Large-scale prevention programming studies.
C   Targeted prevention programs.
D   Health education efforts.

32 Key informants are people

A   Used by law enforcement to provide essential information for arrests.
B   Who are used by program evaluators to monitor program implementation covertly.
C   Who go undercover to provide school officials with tips on drug traffic.
D   Who are essential information sources in needs assessments.

33 What question should be asked at the HIGHEST level of prevention evaluation?

A   Did community-wide behaviors change?
B   Did participants show up?
C   Did program participants' behavior change?
D   Did participants' attitudes change or did self-esteem improve?

34 Including demographic information for outcome program evaluation will help determine if the

A   Program is effective for minority groups.
B   Program is effective for children.
C   Test is valid.
D   Program is effective for different types of participants.

35 Your argument that your program is effective may be strengthened considerably if self-reported change is

A   Matched with demographic data.
B   Recorded on tape.
C   Substantiated by a psychologist.
D   Supplemented by measures collected independently of the program.

36 Focus groups are used to bring together people

A   With common characteristics for implementing programs.
B   From diverse backgrounds to discuss a wide variety of topics.
C   To evaluate the types of proposed program materials.
D   With common characteristics for the needs assessment.

37 An example of an output measure would be

A   A change in the participant's use of a substance.
B   Number of program participants served.
C   An improvement in DUI rates.
D   Pre/Post-tests.

38 Advantages of an internal evaluation are

A   Considered more objective than an external evaluation.
B   Less costly.
C   Involves fewer individuals.
D   Findings are generally considered more credible.

39 After planned data collection is completed, you would then

A   Analyze the data.
B   Prepare a report.
C   Determine stakeholders' needs.
D   None of the above.

40 Archival data is

A   Information from a large number of individuals.
B   Agency compiled information.
C   Hard to find.
D   Collected from surveys.

41 Qualitative data can involve

A   Observations.
B   Document reviews.
C   Measuring people's perceptions.
D   All of the above.

42 The most rigorous evaluation design

A   Utilizes random assignment of participants.
B   Tracks individual for long periods of time after completing program services.
C   Involves multiple data collection procedures.
D   In-depth interviews of program participants.

43 A process evaluation

   A   Is done at the completion of the program.
   B   Is done throughout the delivery of program services.
   C   Involves random assignment of participants.
   D   Involves the collection of participant information after they leave the program.

44 Conducting background checks on prospective volunteers for a prevention program would be an example of demonstrating which principle?

   A   Confidentiality.
   B   Nondiscrimination.
   C   Integrity.
   D   Competence.

45 What is one basic guiding ethical principle in prevention work?

   A   Do no harm.
   B   Lead by example.
   C   Never encourage substance use.
   D   Take every opportunity to spread the prevention message.

46 Regulation that control availability can be implemented by

   A   Local government.
   B   Private organizations such as convenience stores or hospitality establishments.
   C   Police departments.
   D   All of the above.

47 What is a social marketing campaign?

   A   A type of prevention strategy that allows for the selection of the best way to reduce use in a community by popular vote.
   B   A prevention strategy that conveys substance misuse messages to a population like commercial advertising.
   C   An environmental prevention program that targets events and gatherings as the places to deliver its message.
   D   An environmental prevention technique that directs behavior through word of mouth.

48 What are the '4Ps' of advertising?

   A   Person, Place, Price, Probability.
   B   Participation, Promotion, Placement, Price.
   C   Product, Price, Place, Promotion.
   D   Pleasing, Positive, Persuasive, Punchy.

49 Which of the following is NOT a step in the process of creating an effective community coalition?

    A   Defining goals and objectives.
    B   Determining staffing, budget, and resources.
    C   Creating an end date for the coalition's work.
    D   Clarifying expectations of the coalition.

Practice Questions, Set 2

1 The Social Learning Theory was developed by

    A   Erik Erikson.
    B   Abraham Maslow.
    C   Albert Bandura.
    D   David Hawkins and Richard Catalano.

2 The CLOSEST description of the Asset Development Model is one that

    A   Incorporates risk and protective factors.
    B   Was developed by the Search Institute and identifies 40 assets.
    C   Focuses only on resiliency factors.
    D   Identifies developmental tasks by various age groupings.

3 An example of an Information Dissemination approach would be

    A   Classroom presentation on the dangers of illegal drugs.
    B   Mass media campaign on methamphetamine addiction.
    C   Server intervention training workshops.
    D   Student assistance programs.

4 A Youth Development Approach is best characterized as

    A   Policies and procedures a youth program can do to promote youth development.
    B   A focus on protective factors.
    C   A focus on adolescent risk factors.
    D   Mentor relationships.

5 The condition that builds resilience to buffer negative effects (e.g., poverty, drug-abusing environment) are called

    A   Support factors.
    B   Universal factors.
    C   Resilient factors.
    D   Protective factors.

6 Which of the following is NOT one of CSAP's six prevention strategies?

    A   Alternative activities.
    B   Community-based processes.

C   Constructive use of time.

D   Environmental approaches.

7   The Prevention Specialist often encounters the following roles, EXCEPT

A   Technical assistance and training.

B   Group facilitation.

C   Community mobilization.

D   Intervention work.

8   Which of the following approaches best reflects the use of an IOM Indicated approach?

A   Classroom presentation on the dangers of illegal drugs.

B   Mass media campaign on methamphetamine addiction.

C   Server intervention training workshops.

D   Student Assistance Programs.

9   Which of the following is NOT an example of a resiliency factor?

A   Ability to obtain positive attention.

B   Desire to achieve.

C   Favorable community.

D   Positive adult role models.

10   An example of an effective environmental approach to substance misuse prevention is

A   School-based curriculum highlighting community risks.

B   Server intervention training.

C   Program serving student drop-outs.

D   Mass media campaign on meth addiction issues.

11   What is a characteristic of materials that cannot be copyrighted?

A   Tangible.

B   Public domain.

C   Original.

D   Minimally creative.

12   Which of the following would NOT be reflective of a culturally competent approach in prevention planning?

A   The organizational staff ensures publications are available in languages spoken in the community.

B   The organizational staff reflects the ethnicity and diversity of the community.

C   The organizational staff experience diversity training.

D   The organizational staff are encouraged to adopt the clothing styles and fashion of the population being served.

13 Your needs assessment process identified a high rate of alcohol consumption problems among adolescent females. You should

    A   Consider a universal prevention approach.
    B   Consider a youth development approach.
    C   Consider a selective prevention approach.
    D   Implement an asset development approach.

14 Common attributes of resilient children include all of the following, EXCEPT

    A   A young person feels he or she has control over 'things that happen to me.'
    B   A young person has low tolerance for dealing with frustration.
    C   A young person experiences caring neighbors and adults they can trust.
    D   A young person places high value on helping others.

15 A way the media can be used to educate and inform is through

    A   Parenting skills classes.
    B   After-school programming.
    C   PTA meetings.
    D   Opinion Editorials.

16 What is the difference between hearing and listening?

    A   Involve them in the planning process.
    B   Ensure food is provided at the planning meeting.
    C   Get a PSA on local television.
    D   Get an announcement placed in the local newspaper.

17 An example of environment in the public health model would be

    A   A professional baseball park.
    B   A public fair, with a restricted area for beer sales.
    C   A bar.
    D   All of the above.

18 To understand the role that media (e.g., advertisements, movies, or songs) can have in shaping adolescent behavior involves which theoretical perspective

    A   Maslow's Hierarchy of Needs.
    B   Bandura's Social Learning Theory.
    C   Erik Erikson's Theory of Development.
    D   None of the above.

19 Product placement strategies are an example of

    A   An Environmental approach.
    B   Information Dissemination approach.

C   Alternative Activity approach.

D   Community-based Process approach.

20 Which of the following is NOT a component of the process model of communication?

A   **Participant**.

B   Noise.

C   Chanel.

D   Sender.

21 Target population analysis is best carried out using

A   Bandura's social learning theory.

B   The IOM model approach.

C   Youth development approach.

D   The CSAP six strategies.

22 The attitude and habit that MOST increases cultural sensitivity is

A   Leading.

B   Demonstrating sympathy.

C   Displaying concern.

D   Working alongside.

23 Can an individual belong to multiple cultures?

A   Yes.

B   No.

C   Only in some situations.

24 Copyright permission is only required for

A   Written materials.

B   Songs.

C   Videotapes.

D   All of the above.

25 What is an example of a price intervention prevention strategy?

A   Surveying retailers on how much they charge for certain alcoholic beverages.

B   Documenting how much money is spent each year on alcohol or tobacco.

C   Increasing the sales tax on alcoholic beverages.

D   Limiting the number of alcoholic beverages that can be purchased at any one time.

26 Which of the following is NOT a step in the process of putting on a social marketing campaign?

A   Evaluation.
B   Define the messages and communication channels.
C   Determine the history of media impact in the community.
D   Develop and pretest or pilot materials.

27 An approach to becoming culturally competent would include

I   Becoming fully aware of one's own cultural history.
II   Becoming aware of how other cultures are portrayed in the media.
III   Acknowledging the historical relationships of one's own cultural background with that of other cultural groups.

A   I and III only.
B   II and III only.
C   III only.
D   All of the above.

28 To be a good facilitator, you must NOT be

A   Flexible.
B   Authoritative.
C   Respectful.
D   Confident.

29 A professional code of ethics generally does not

A   Promote high standards on the job.
B   Create a set of benchmarks to evaluate job performance.
C   Provide guidance per acceptable kinds of behavior.
D   Specify appropriate client behaviors.

30 In your role as a facilitator and Prevention Specialist, you would NOT

A   Select the prevention program approach for them.
B   Assure a neutral position in a heated discussion.
C   Make eye contact, as this is disrespectful.
D   Summarize points, as this is boring.

31 In order to increase diverse community involvement in a coalition, you should

A   Present at the schools in the target communities.
B   Use flyers in the desired communities.
C   Use public events (e.g., fairs) to advertise your needs.
D   Get coalition members to go directly to their targeted community and recruit potential members.

Answer Key - Test 1

1. A	6. A	11. A	16. D	21. D	26. B	31. C	36. D	41. D	46. D
2. B	7. B	12. D	17. B	22. B	27. A	32. D	37. B	42. A	47. B
3. D	8. D	13. C	18. B	23. A	28. C	33. A	38. B	43. B	48. C
4. D	9. D	14. C	19. D	24. B	29. A	34. D	39. A	44. D	49. C
5. B	10. A	15. B	20. A	25. D	30. B	35. D	40. B	45. A	

Answer Key - Test 2

1. C	6. C	11. B	16. A	21. B	26. C	31. D
2. B	7. D	12. D	17. D	22. D	27. D	
3. B	8. D	13. C	18. B	23. A	28. B	
4. A	9. C	14. B	19. A	24. D	29. D	
5. D	10. B	15. D	20. F	25. C	30. A	

10 Understanding the Correct Answer

When studying for the exam, I have found it most helpful to thoroughly review any practice test questions I could find. You want to be able to articulate *why* a certain answer is the best choice. It is recommended that you first complete the practice tests in the previous chapter and then review the content of this chapter, which provides an in-depth explanation for the correct answer and should help you in understanding any auxiliary topics connected to the test question. If you've created a study group, consider a walkthrough of this chapter together and discuss each question. As a general test-taking tip, first eliminate the answer choices you know to be untrue. Often you will find it fairly easy to choose the best answer from what remains. If you get stuck, be sure to reach out to your professional network and start a conversation. Your knowledge of these concepts is foundational to your ability to operate with the highest competency as a prevention professional and will be of great help to you when taking the examination.

Practice Questions and Answers, Set 1

1   A needs assessment that uses information collected from interviews, focus groups, and/or observations involving document reviews to produce a descriptive report is called

    A   **Qualitative data.**
    B   Outcome data.
    C   Quantitative data.
    D   Indicator data.

It is important to have a clear understanding of key terms related to evaluation. *Qualitative data* is descriptive data that provides in-depth information on the subject of interest. This means conducting interviews, hosting focus groups, and any other activities that yield descriptive data. In answering this question, you should also know the definitions of the other terms. This will help you eliminate answer choices.

Outcome data – focused on data that shows how the participants' lives were changed or affected by the program activities.

DOI: 10.4324/9781003053941-13

Quantitative data – focused on describing an issue numerically, usually involved conduction surveys.

Indicator data – focused on helping us measure program progress and effectiveness.

2   One of the goals of prevention is to learn about the long-term effects on our culture. The type of assessment needed to measure these effects is called

   A   Outcome Assessment.
   B   **Cultural Diversity Assessment**.
   C   Process Assessment.
   D   Long-Term Assessment.

You should be able to immediately eliminate options A, C, and D. Answers A and D are focused on measuring the outcomes of a prevention program. Answer C will provide you with information on how the program operated.

3   Theories of causation help identify why youth begin using drugs. substance misuse prevention program designers must determine what factors are involved. At the most basic level these factors are

   A   Schools and communities.
   B   Family and peers.
   C   Individuals and family.
   D   **Risk and protective.**

Answer choices A, B, and C represent the five domains of influence under the risk and protective factors concept. This leaves option D as the only possible answer.

4   It is important to match risk and protective factors in substance misuse prevention programming. Which of the following statements have a good match between risk and protective factors and programming?

   I   *A school-based program working on self-esteem with children who live in abusive families.*
  II   *A school-based program working on life skills with low-risk students.*
 III   *A school-based support group program for students who have violated school substance policies.*

   A   I only.
   B   III only.
   C   I and II only.
   D   **II and III only.**

In this question, you're looking at the match between the intervention approach and the characteristics of the audience served. Option 'I' seems the most inappropriate match: self-esteem programming for children living in an abusive home. If you recall, our prevention code of ethics would require us to report knowledge of such a living situation. Therefore this option would trigger for those children to receive a higher level of care than what we would provide as a prevention specialist. Based on this understanding, you can eliminate answer choices A and C. The only thing left to decide is if there's an appropriate match for options II and III. Option II describes a universal population and Option II describes an indicated population.

5   Media campaigns dealing with prevention techniques affect audiences by

   A   Educating the public.
   B   **Increasing problem awareness.**
   C   Changing attitudes toward the behavior.
   D   Changing the behavior.

When you think about the CSAP 6 prevention strategies you will quickly see why you can eliminate answer choices A, C, and D. These answer choices all deal with strategies more intensive than a media campaign. However, you can successfully increase awareness of the problem by using a media campaign.

6   Targeted programs are

   A   **High-impact, highly focused programs for risk reduction.**
   B   Low-impact, broadly publicized programs for interdiction.
   C   High-impact, broadly publicized programs for intervention.
   D   Programs funded for a short time to serve a specific group.

You can eliminate choices B and C because they are both focused 'broadly,' which is the opposite of 'targeted.' We are able to eliminate answer D because there is no time limitation on a target program.

7   The best description of the 40 Developmental Assets Model is

   A   Helps prevent risky behaviors in youth.
   B   **Developed by the Search Institute and focuses on strengths needed for success.**
   C   Is based on resiliency only.
   D   Looks at the strengths of each person.

Answer choice B most comprehensively defines the 40 Developmental Assets. You should easily be able to recall that this concept was created by the Search Institute in the 1990s.

8   A thorough prevention needs assessment process should involve

   I   *Key stakeholders.*
   II   *Collection of consumption/consequence data.*

III *Funding options.*
IV *Identification of target (affected) populations.*

    A   I only.
    B   III only.
    C   I and IV only.
    D   **I, II, and IV only.**

The discovery of funding options is not a prevention needs assessment task. Stakeholders, the collection of consumption/consequence data, and the identification of the affected population are all key components.

9   The Strategic Prevention Framework is used to

    I   *Prepare a needs assessment.*
   II   *Identify community resources.*
  III   *Build capacity.*
  IV   *Select and implement an appropriate prevention approach.*

    A   I only.
    B   I and II only.
    C   III and IV only.
    D   **I, II, III, and IV.**

The Strategic Prevention Framework (SPF) has five foundation components: assessment, capacity, planning, implementation, and evaluation. All of the activities listed are foundational to using the Strategic Prevention Framework.

10   The IOM health care model defines three types of prevention approaches/target populations. The terminology that BEST reflects one of these types is

    A   **Universal.**
    B   Children of Substance Abusing Parents (COSAP).
    C   High-Risk Youth.
    D   Substance Users.

The IOM model has three levels: universal, selective, and indicated; making choice A the only possible answer.

11   An example of an indicated prevention strategy includes

    A   **Student Assistance Program (SAP).**
    B   Media Campaign.
    C   Schools Assemblies.
    D   Social Norm Program.

Indicated prevention strategies are dedicated to providing service for the highest risk level and require a targeted approach. Student assistance programs are designed to provide services and support for the removal of barriers to learning for the student. Answer choices B, C, and D do not meet this standard and would be considered an inappropriate intervention match for an indicated audience.

12   The most important feature in creating a logic model is

A   They try out multiple strategies.
B   They enhance community involvement.
C   They help you determine appropriate staffing patterns.
D   **They connect your outcomes and your goals.**

Logic models are fundamentally used to connect your program activities to your anticipated outcomes for the populations served.

13   The prevention planning structure using a five-step process that includes assessment, capacity, planning, implementation, and evaluation is known as

A   Problem Identification and Referral Model.
B   Social Development Strategy Model.
C   **Strategic Prevention Framework.**
D   Public Health Model.

This question clearly defines the first-step process of SPF. Option A is one of the CSAP 6 Strategies. Option B is a human behavior model and not a prevention planning structure. Option D has just three main components: host, environment, agent.

14   Mobilizing community members to participate in a community prevention effort is an example of

A   Community readiness.
B   Problem prioritization.
C   **Coalition building.**
D   Community needs assessment.

You can eliminate options B and D, as they do not relate to community mobilization. You might be tempted to choose option A. However, community readiness is an assessment strategy that provides you with information on the community's consciousness concerning the substance misuse problem.

15   You are planning to use a proven, evidence-based program, but realize it is not feasible to implement all of the program components. You should

A   Not proceed at all with your choice.
B   **Consult with the developers to determine potential impact.**

C   Go ahead, as most programs can be modified to meet local circumstances.

D   Add additional alternatives to fill out the missing components.

This is actually one of my favorite concepts to understand. Prevention is a science and therefore programs are designed with intention and purpose. You should always consult with the developer when you want to make modifications to how a program is delivered.

16   A prevention program that has been designated as a best practice means

A   It has been adapted by many prevention programs throughout the country.

B   It reflects the specific cultural needs of the community.

C   It needs to involve a skilled, experienced program director.

D   **It has been shown through research and evaluation to be effective.**

Although options A, B, and C are often true characteristics of a best practice, a program becomes a best practice through the research and evaluation of the practice showing it to be an effective strategy.

17   What is the best way to engage community members?

A   Ask them for their advice.

B   **Get them involved in the planning process.**

C   Survey them.

D   Conduct a focus group.

Community engagement is critical to the success of prevention programs, and the best way to engage community members is to invite them to the table! So often we only reach out to the community for options A, C, and D. This creates the dynamic that the community is just a source of information and not a co-creator in developing solutions. Our goal as prevention professionals is not to be the 'savior,' yet to be an advocate in helping leverage the science of prevention to improve community health outcomes.

18   What level of networking and collaboration best describes the following situation?

At a meeting, various after-school programs share their summer schedule with each other.

A   Coordination.

B   **Communication/Networking.**

C   Cooperation.

D   Collaboration.

This question is best answered by knowing the definitions of the various levels of networking

- Communication/Networking – mutual sharing of information
- Cooperation – mutual support of activities without a formal agreement
- Coordination – mutual planning of activities and even modifying events to benefit the whole
- Collaboration – formal agreements in place and the shared development of strategic goals

19 If your community coalition lacks participation from a specific cultural group you should

A Go with the group that has volunteered to serve in your coalition.
B Invite them to your next planning meeting.
C Wait until the current coalition is completed with its work.
D **Have collation members go to their community and ask them to participate.**

The members of the coalition are your most valuable asset. You should not carry the mantel of the coalition work. The members should be actively involved in the recruitment and retention of members. It is through the collective action of the members that prevention initiatives are most successful.

20 In selecting a prevention program, what should you do?

A **Select the program with community input.**
B Base decision on what other prevention programs are doing.
C Base selection on the prevention literature.
D Select a universal-based approach.

Remember from question 17, we've established the need for the community to be engaged in the planning process. By this same logic, we also understand the importance of the community being engaged in the selection of the prevention program. Option B can be eliminated because we shouldn't do things just because of what others are doing. You might be tempted to choose Option C, however, it's inherently implied that you used prevention literature to curate the list of appropriate interventions for the community to select from. Option D is not relevant, because you don't have enough information to know if a universal approach is appropriate.

21 A community is in denial when it

A Does not recognize it has a substance problem.
B Has no active leaders interested in the problem.
C Has not engaged in the collection and analysis of substance data.
D **All of the above.**

A strong knowledge of the stages of community readiness will make this question easy to answer. A community in denial will be passive and guarded, and there will be little or no recognition that a substance problem exists.

22   One of the most effective strategies to use involves scare tactics, presenting the realities associated with substance use.

A   True.
B   **False.**

Scare tactics are from before our field had an evolution in thought. There was a time in history when we believed that fear-based learning was effective. Although there now exists a body of research that shows such tactics as ineffective, we still see remnants of the strategy in society.

23   A prevention strategy aimed at informing broad segments of society is called a

A   **Universal program.**
B   Selected program.
C   Indicated program.
D   Risk and protective approach

Answer choice D can be eliminated as the choice is not relevant to the question. The risk and protective approach focus on the conditions that increase or decrease the likelihood of experiencing positive or negative life experiences. In question 10, we identified the three types of IOM audiences. Answers B and C are aimed at a targeted audience.

24   A program that has been researched and found to be effective is known as

A   Proven.
B   **Best Practice.**
C   Promising.
D   Excellent.

The question is straightforward. The definition of a 'best practice' is a program that has been researched and found to be effective. You can eliminate options A and D as neither of these terms represents a program that has been 'researched and found to be effective.' That leaves us with the 'promising' option, which by definition means we do not yet have enough research to call it a 'best practice.'

25   Ways you might encourage community readiness to address their local substance problem include

A   Provide educational outreach to community leaders.
B   Provide prevalence rates on substance problems.
C   Conduct in-service training.
D   **All of the above.**

The first step in improving community readiness is to increase awareness of the substance problem. All three options will help accomplish this goal, and therefore answer D is the best.

26 A goal statement

    A   Specifies what and when something is to be accomplished.
    B   **Is general and inclusive.**
    C   Identifies who will do what tasks.
    D   Is the same as a mission statement.

Your goal statement is the 'pie in the sky' and therefore is general and inclusive. Every other answer choice for this question is too specific to be a goal statement. In fact, answer choices A, C, and D are items that would be a part of your action plan.

27 An objective statement

    A   **Is time-specific and measurable.**
    B   Identifies specific individuals and their responsibilities.
    C   Is general and inclusive.
    D   Compares planned to achieved tasks.

Unlike the goal statement, our objectives should be SMART – specific, measurable, attainable, realistic, and time-bound. Answer choice A is the clear choice for this question.

28 A community readiness process

    A   Identifies community resources available for prevention activities.
    B   Summarizes substance use and problems associated with their use.
    C   **Determines whether community members believe they have a substance problem or not.**
    D   All of the above.

Answer choices A and B describe the community needs assessment process. Community readiness is focused on understanding the community's perception of the local substance use issues.

29 Consumption data is generally derived from

    A   **Surveys.**
    B   Key informant interviews.
    C   Prevention program records.
    D   Focus groups.

Although there are many ways to collect consumption data, this question is looking for the most general way that data is gathered. Surveys are the go-to method for making statements about the consumption patterns in a particular community.

30 A gap analysis refers to

A   The difference in consumption patterns between adolescent youths from different age groupings.

B   **The differences in available community resources as compared to the extent of the substance problems.**

C   The number of current prevention programs as compared to the number of services available in prior years.

D   The difference in funding allocations for current prevention efforts as compared to the funding amount one year ago.

During the capacity stage of prevention planning, we should have conducted a community asset map. The asset map will show you the resources in the community that can be leveraged to accomplish the intended program goal. It is at this point that you are able to establish a gap analysis, which creates a relationship between the problem identified during the needs assessment and the community resources currently available to address that need. Ideally, the prevention program being designed should address the 'gap' as a means of improving the health outcomes for the community served.

31 The greatest optimism in the development of substance misuse prevention activities has come from

A   Individualized prevention efforts.
B   Large-scale prevention programming studies.
C   **Targeted prevention programs.**
D   Health education efforts.

The reason the IOM categories exist is to assist prevention programs in being appropriate for the audience. Targeted programs are most effective because these programs are specialized in their intention and there is a clear match between the audience's risk and protective factors and the intervention strategy being used.

32 Key informants are people

A   Used by law enforcement to provide essential information for arrests.
B   Who are used by program evaluators to monitor program implementation covertly.
C   Who go undercover to provide school officials with tips on drug traffic.
D   **Who are essential information sources in needs assessments.**

Answer choice D is the definition of a key informant, no other choice is possible. Key informant interviews are a type of data source when doing a needs assessment. Key informants provide us with qualitative data.

33 What question should be asked at the HIGHEST level of prevention evaluation?

    A **Did community-wide behaviors change?**
    B Did participants show up?
    C Did program participants' behavior change?
    D Did participants' attitudes change or did self-esteem improve?

Think of the logic model. Our goal statement is our highest level of evaluation and this statement should be general and broad. This means looking at if community-wide changes occurred as a result of the prevention intervention. Answer choice B is a process evaluation question. Answer choice C is an intermediate evaluation question and Answer choice D is a short-term evaluation question. Remember attitudes must change before behavior can change.

34 Including demographic information for outcome program evaluation will help determine if the

    A Program is effective for minority groups.
    B Program is effective for children.
    C Test is valid.
    D **Program is effective for different types of participants.**

Collecting demographic information provides valuable insight to the process evaluation. So often demographic information is collected as a checkbox for establishing the degree of diversity in the community served. Demographic information helps in understanding how different participants respond to an intervention and can help you in discovering the need for adaptations. It's important to remember that demographics include a wide variety of characteristics: gender, race, age, geography, religion, education, etc.

35 Your argument that your program is effective may be strengthened considerably if self-reported change is

    A Matched with demographic data.
    B Recorded on tape.
    C Substantiated by a psychologist.
    D **Supplemented by measures collected independently of the program.**

Third-party data that supports your claim of an effective program is the gold standard for establishing a program as either promising or a best practice.

36 Focus groups are used to bring together people

    A With common characteristics for implementing programs.
    B From diverse backgrounds to discuss a wide variety of topics.

C   To evaluate the types of proposed program materials.
D   **With common characteristics for needs assessment.**

Focus groups are used to help us better understand a specific concept. For example, let's say you have data showing underage drinking is an issue in your community and you want to know more about why and how the youth are getting access to alcohol. You conduct a focus group with youth to gain some insight on this specific issue.

37   An example of an output measure would be

A   A change in the participant's use of a substance.
B   **Number of program participants served.**
C   An improvement in DUI rates.
D   Pre/Posttests

Think back to your knowledge of logic models. Outputs count the program activities such as the number of sessions, participants, trainings, etc. Answers A and D would be types of outcome data. Pre/posttests are a type of data collection instrument, where you provide a pretest before the program starts and then conduct a posttest after the program ends.

38   Advantages with an internal evaluation are

A   Considered more objective than an external evaluation.
B   **Less costly.**
C   Involves fewer individuals.
D   Findings are generally considered more credible.

We can immediately remove options A and D as false statements. External evaluations are objective and often more credible than an internal eva-luation. We can also eliminate answer choice C, as there's no guarantee that an internal evaluation would involve fewer people than an external evaluation.

39   After planned data collection is completed, you would then

A   **Analyze the data.**
B   Prepare a report.
C   Determine stakeholders' needs.
D   None of the above.

The next logical step after collecting data is the analyze that data, so you can better understand the community problem.

40   Archival data is

A   Information from a large number of individuals.
B   **Agency compiled information.**

C   Hard to find.
D   Collected from surveys.

Archival data is collected and stored by someone else; typically a county health department, foundation, or some other type of agency. Interestingly with this question, the other answer choices can also be a true statement about archival data. However, they are not the ONLY true statement. Answer choice B is the only statement that can stand alone as true.

41   Qualitative data can involve

A   Observations.
B   Document reviews.
C   Measuring people's perceptions.
D   **All of the above.**

Qualitative data is not easily reduced to numbers, therefore answer choices A, B, and C are data collection methods that call under qualitative.

42   The most rigorous evaluation design

A   **Utilizes random assignment of participants.**
B   Tracks individual for long periods of time after completing program services.
C   Involves multiple data collection procedures.
D   In-depth interviews of program participants.

Random assignment of participants is the gold standard for a program design. This design uses sophisticated methods to reduce bias in the program design. Reducing bias is what helps us make bold statements about 'what works.' Answer B, C, and D are all strong evaluation methods, however, this question asks for the 'most rigorous' design.

43   A process evaluation

A   Is done at the completion of the program.
B   **Is done throughout the delivery of program services.**
C   Involves random assignment of participants.
D   Involves the collection of participant information after they leave the program.

The process evaluation is focused on what was done during the program. This information helps us understand how we achieved certain outcomes.

44   Conducting background checks on prospective volunteers for a prevention program would be an example of demonstrating which principle?

A   Confidentiality
B   Nondiscrimination

C   Integrity
D   **Competence**

You can use a process of elimination to answer this question. We can get rid of answer choices A and B, just because confidentiality and non-discrimination are not connected to why we do background checks. Integrity is focused on how we operate 'on the job.' Background checks are conducted before a volunteer is allowed to assist with program activities. Background checks include the review of all the information gathered to ensure the person is properly vetted and capable of providing quality service.

45   What is one basic guiding ethical principle in prevention work?

A   **Do no harm.**
B   Lead by example.
C   Never encourage substance use.
D   Take every opportunity to spread the prevention message.

46   Regulation that control availability can be implemented by

A   Local government.
B   Private organizations such as convenience stores or hospitality establishments.
C   Police departments.
D   **All of the above.**

Controlling the availability of a substance is a strong environmental strategy. It can use employed by any of the agencies listed for this question.

47   What is a social marketing campaign?

A   A type of prevention strategy that allows for the selection of the best way to reduce use in a community by popular vote.
B   **A prevention strategy that conveys substance misuse messages to a population like commercial advertising.**
C   An environmental prevention program that targets events and gatherings as the places to deliver its message.
D   An environmental prevention technique that directs behavior through word of mouth.

A social marketing campaign leverages media to raise awareness about substance misuse issues. Answer choice A can be eliminated because it is describing a decision-making process. Neither answer choices C or D accurately describe a social marketing campaign. Social marketing campaigns are not limited to specific events or word-of-mouth. communication.

48 What are the '4Ps' of advertising?

A   Person, Place, Price, Probability.
B   Participation, Promotion, Placement, Price.
C   **Product, Price, Place, Promotion.**
D   Pleasing, Positive, Persuasive, Punchy.

This question is easily answered by having the 4Ps memorized.

49 Which of the following is NOT a step in the process of creating an effective community coalition?

A   Defining goals and objectives.
B   Determining staffing, budget, and resources.
C   **Creating an end date for the coalition's work.**
D   Clarifying expectations of the coalition.

Answer choices A, B, and D are easily identified as important steps in creating a coalition. Creating an end date for the coalition's work is not a necessary step. In fact, what most coalitions experience is a never-ending source of community substance use issues that could be addressed through the collective action of a coalition.

Practice Questions and Answers, Set 2

1   The Social Learning Theory was developed by

A   Erik Erikson.
B   Abraham Maslow.
C   **Albert Bandura.**
D   David Hawkins and Richard Catalano.

This question is easily answered when you have memorized the main theories that guide prevention practice. Erik Erikson is responsible for the stages of development. Abraham Maslow introduced the hierarchy of needs. Hawkins & Catalano introduced the concepts of risk and protective factors.

2   Which of the following is NOT a leadership style?

A   Problem Solver
B   **Discusser**
C   Director
D   Developer

There are four primary leadership styles: director, developer, problem solver, and delegator. Having these memorized will assist you in answering any questions related to leadership styles.

3   An example of an Information Dissemination approach would be

   A   Classroom presentation on the dangers of illegal drugs.
   B   **Mass media campaign on methamphetamine addiction.**
   C   Server intervention training workshops.
   D   Student Assistance Programs.

This question taps into your understanding of the CSAP 6 strategies. Answer choices A and C are a prevention education approach. Answer choice D is a problem identification and referral strategy. Information dissemination approach focuses on one-way communication.

4   A Youth Development Approach is best characterized as

   A   **Policies and procedures a youth program can do to promote youth development.**
   B   A focus on protective factors.
   C   A focus on adolescent risk factors.
   D   Mentor relationships.

A youth development approach would include components from four answer choices. Option A is the best and most comprehensive choice.

5   The condition that builds resilience to buffer negative effects (e.g., poverty, drug-abusing environment) are called

   A   Support Factors.
   B   Universal Factors.
   C   Resilient Factors.
   D   **Protective Factors.**

You may have been tempted to choose Answer choice C. However, this question tests your knowledge of risk and protective factors. The resilience approach is focused on the complex process of understanding how an individual thrives despite the environment. The risk and protective factors theory is a predictive theory, meaning it empirically states if certain conditions are present, a probable outcome may result.

6   Which of the following is NOT one of CSAP's six prevention strategies?

   A   Alternative Activities.
   B   Community-Based Processes.
   C   **Constructive Use of Time.**
   D   Environmental Approaches.

You should be able to easily names the CSAP 6 strategies, which helps you quickly answer this question. Additionally, when you are familiar with the 40 Development Assets, you will identify Answer choice C as an external asset.

7 The Prevention Specialist often encounters the following roles, EXCEPT

  A Technical assistance and training.
  B Group facilitation.
  C Community mobilization.
  D **Intervention work.**

As a Prevention Specialist, you will regularly provide technical assistance, training, group facilitation, and community mobilizing activities. This only leaves Answer choice D as the mobe obvious 'exception.' We often use the word 'intervention' to describe a specific prevention approach. In this instance, 'intervention' work is used to describe the strategy designed to convince someone to enter into treatment. This requires specialized skills and is outside of our scope of work. Our CSAP strategy of problem identification and referral to treatment is NOT intervention work.

8 Which of the following approaches best reflects the use of an IOM Indicated approach?

  A Classroom presentation on the dangers of illegal drugs.
  B Mass media campaign on methamphetamine addiction.
  C Server intervention training workshops.
  D **Student Assistance Programs.**

The Indicated approach focuses on the audience with the highest risk in an attempt to prevent the onset of a substance use disorder. This is our most targeted approach to prevention practice.

9 Which of the following is NOT an example of a resiliency factor?

  A Ability to obtain positive attention.
  B Desire to achieve.
  C **Favorable community.**
  D Positive adult role models.

10 An example of an effective environmental approach to substance misuse prevention is

  A School-based curriculum highlighting community risks.
  B **Server intervention training.**
  C Program serving student drop-outs.
  D Mass media campaign on meth addiction issues.

Environmental strategies are designed to create changes in the community conditions that perpetuate substance use disorders. Server training is twofold in nature. The approach addresses social access by training servers to properly check for the age of anyone they serve. Additionally, servers are trained to recognize signs of intoxication and liabilities connected to overserving customers.

11   What is a characteristic of materials that cannot be copyrighted?

    A   Tangible.
    B   **Public domain.**
    C   Original
    D   Minimally creative.

This question deals with professional ethics and is easily answered when you understand the definition of public domain. Public domain content is not owned by a specific person or entity. This happens for a few reasons: the content existed before copyright was created, the copyright terms have expired, or have been suspended for some reason.

12   Which of the following would NOT be reflective of a culturally competent approach in prevention planning?

    A   The organizational staff ensures publications are available in languages spoken in the community.
    B   The organizational staff reflects the ethnicity and diversity of the community.
    C   The organizational staff experience diversity training.
    D   **The organizational staff are encouraged to adopt the clothing styles and fashion of the population being served.**

Answer choices A, B, and C demonstrate a culturally competent organization. However, Answer choice D does not align with being culturally responsive to a communities needs, and depending on the community could be viewed as an offensive act.

13   Your needs assessment process identified a high rate of alcohol consumption problems among adolescent females. You should

    A   Consider a universal prevention approach.
    B   Consider a youth development approach.
    C   **Consider a selective prevention approach.**
    D   Implement an asset development approach.

The data identified a risk factor linked to membership in a specific group (adolescent females). This is the definition of a selective prevention approach. Remember, universal approaches are not targeted to a specific audience.

14   Common attributes of resilient children include all of the following, EXCEPT

    A   A young person feels he or she has control over 'things that happen to me.'
    B   **A young person has a low tolerance for dealing with frustration.**

    C   A young person experiences caring neighbors and adults they can trust.

    D   A young person places high value on helping others.

With this question, you are looking for the option that does not define resilience. As you review choices A, C, and D it should be easy to see how these attributes would contribute to a young person's resilience.

15   A way the media can be used to educate and inform is through

    A   Parenting skills classes.

    B   After-school programming.

    C   PTA meetings.

    D   **Opinion Editorials.**

Answer choice D is the only media example amongst the four choices, making this an easy process of elimination question. Additionally, you should recognize: Answer choice A as a prevention education strategy, Answer choice B could be a prevention education and/or alternative activity approach, and Answer choice C as an irrelevant topic for the question.

16   What is the difference between hearing and listening?

    A   **Hearing is receiving sound waves, while listening is processing the information conveyed.**

    B   Listening and hearing cannot occur at the same time.

    C   Listening is passive, while hearing is active.

    D   Hearing happens individually, while listening occurs in a pair or group.

Hearing is the technical term for what happens as sounds waves enter the ear. It is through listening (which is an active process) that we interpret what has been heard by our ears.

17   An example of the environment in the public health model would be

    A   A professional baseball park.

    B   A public fair, with a restricted area for beer sales.

    C   A bar.

    D   **All of the above.**

Think back to the three components of the public health model: agent, host, and environment. The environment is the setting in which substance use issues occur. This setting can be favorable or unfavorable. All three answer choices are examples of 'environments' where substance use can occur in a community.

18   To understand the role that media (e.g., advertisements, movies, or songs) can have in shaping adolescent behavior involves which theoretical perspective

    A   Maslow's Hierarchy of Needs.

    B   **Bandura's Social Learning Theory.**

    C   Erik Erikson's Theory of Development.

    D   None of the above.

Bandura's theory is that learning occurs through modeling others and that this behavior is either encouraged or discouraged by the consequences the individual experiences. This theory is used to understand how the media can provide youth with behaviors to model. Teaching media literacy is one of the many ways we address the issue of youth modeling the behaviors that are counterproductive reducing substance use disorders.

19   Product placement strategies are an example of

    A   **An Environmental approach.**

    B   Information Dissemination approach.

    C   Alternative Activity approach.

    D   Community-based Process approach.

If you're unsure about this question, an easy process of elimination is to define all the terms. Answer B is focused on our one-way community strategies. Answer C is the supplemental activities we use to complement other prevention approaches. Answer D focuses on the set of strategies that help a community provide better behavioral health services.

20   Which of the following is NOT a component of the process model of communication?

    A   **Participant**

    B   Noise

    C   Chanel

    D   Sender

In the process model of community, we use the language of receiver not participant. There are senders and receivers of communication messages.

21   Target population analysis is best carried out using

    A   Bandura's social learning theory.

    B   **The IOM model approach.**

    C   Youth development approach.

    D   The CSAP six strategies.

The IOM categories help us identify the characteristics of the population. No other answer choice is focused on a target population analysis.

22   The attitude and habit that MOST increases cultural sensitivity is

    A   Leading.

    B   Demonstrating sympathy.

C   Displaying concern.
D   **Working alongside.**

Being culturally sensitive means working alongside communities. We assist them in understanding, planning, implementing, and evaluating substance prevention programs. The community is the expert in their own culture. We are not there to lead them, yet we exist to help uncover the assets already in the community that can be leveraged to create positive change.

23   Can an individual belong to multiple cultures?

A   **Yes.**
B   No.
C   Only in some situations.

We all belong to multiple cultures! Culture is life and includes many dimensions: age, gender, religion, geography, language, ethnicity, social habits, music, food, and so much more!

24   Copyright permission is only required for

A   Written materials.
B   Songs.
C   Videotapes.
D   **All of the above.**

Copyright permission is required for any materials that are not your own. Permission gives you the legal right to use someone else's creative content. Be sure to give credit when using content from someone else's work.

25   What is an example of a price intervention prevention strategy?

A   Surveying retailers on how much they charge for certain alcoholic beverages.
B   Documenting how much money is spent each year on alcohol or tobacco.
C   **Increasing the sales tax on alcoholic beverages.**
D   Limiting the number of alcoholic beverages that can be purchased at any one time.

Price interventions are an environmental approach that focuses on increasing the 'cost' by raising taxes on those items. Answer choices A, B, and D do not meet the definition of a price intervention.

26   Which of the following is NOT a step in the process of putting on a social marketing campaign?

A   Evaluation.
B   Define the messages and communication channels.

C   **Determine the history of media impact in the community.**

D   Develop and pretest or pilot materials.

Although learning about the history of media impact on the community is helpful information, it is not a step in the process of putting together a social marketing campaign.

27   An approach to becoming culturally competent would include

I   Becoming fully aware of one's own cultural history.

II   Becoming aware of how other cultures are portrayed in the media.

III   Acknowledging the historical relationships of one's own cultural background with that of other cultural groups.

A   I and III only.
B   II and III only.
C   III only.
D   **All of the above.**

Developing a sense of cultural intelligence requires us to start with a personal evaluation of our own cultural identity. We also should reflect on how the media has played a role in our perception of other cultures. This will help in identifying any biases. Without the knowledge of our own biases, how can we truly operate in a culturally intelligent way? Lastly, we should also reflect on historical relationships between various cultures. We are an accumulation of the past, which means we as a society carry the trauma of the past. Knowledge of this trauma helps us work alongside communities to advocate for equity and improve community resilience.

28   To be a good facilitator, you must NOT be

A   Flexible.
B   **Authoritative.**
C   Respectful.
D   Confident.

Being authoritative is often counterproductive to the goal of a facilitator. As a facilitator, you create an environment where ideas are welcome. This means being flexible, respectful, and confident.

29   A professional code of ethics generally does not

A   Promote high standards on the job.
B   Create a set of benchmarks to evaluate job performance.
C   Provide guidance per acceptable kinds of behavior.
D   **Specify appropriate participant behaviors.**

Our professional code of ethics focuses on OUR professional behavior. There is typically a separate document that outlines expectations for participants (ground rules, participant code of conduct, etc.).

30 In your role as a facilitator and Prevention Specialist, you would NOT

A **Select the prevention program approach for them.**
B Assure a neutral position in a heated discussion.
C Make eye contact, as this is disrespectful.
D Summarize points, as this is boring.

Our job is to work alongside the community. Selecting the prevention approach without community input is not a best practice. Answer choices B, C, and D are all false. As a facilitator, you will mediate heated discussions. Eye contact increases your appearance of confidence, and you should only be avoided in specific cultural situations where eye contact is considered disrespectful. Finally, summarizing the points discussed will ensure everyone is on the same page.

31 In order to increase diverse community involvement in a coalition, you should

A Present at the schools in the target communities.
B Use flyers in the desired communities.
C Use public events (e.g., fairs) to advertise your needs.
D **Get coalition members to go directly to their targeted community and recruit potential members.**

The best way to increase the diversity of your coalition is by having the current members recruit others. Remember coalition work is done through collection action and you as the Prevention Specialist should not be doing all the work.

11 Glossary of Terms

Abraham Maslow
Created Maslow's Hierarchy of Needs, which suggests that as humans' basic needs are met, they become more motivated to achieve higher levels of motivation.

ACEs
Adverse Childhood Experiences. The ACEs questionnaire has 10 questions and is separated into four types of experiences: emotional, physical, sexual abuse, and witnessing violence between parents or caregivers.

Accommodation
A concept from Piaget's Cognitive Developmental Stages Theory. The process of change one's thinking when new information does fit into an existing schema.

Adaptation
The skilled prevention professional considers the needs of a community when developing a program, which often requires adaptations to the original curriculum. Adaptation does NOT take away from the curriculum. It is advised to contact the developer before making any adaptations.

Addiction
Compulsion and a craving to use alcohol or other drugs regardless of negative or adverse consequences. Addiction is characterized by psychological dependence, and often (depending on the drug or drugs) physical dependence. An inability to set or maintain limits, resulting in loss of control, is also a characteristic of addiction. Addiction is the most severe form of substance use disorder and is classified as a chronic brain disease that has the potential for recurrence and recovery.

Advocacy
Advocacy is the use of the political process to influence laws, regulations, and policies. Advocacy may include creating petitions, writing letters, making phone calls, and going door-to-door in your community. It's important to realize the difference between lobbying and advocating because you can lose funding if there is any suspicion of crossing the line.

DOI: 10.4324/9781003053941-14

Agent

In the public health model, the agent is the AOD substance of concern causing harm to the individual (e.g., tobacco, alcohol, other drugs). The 'agent' acts directly on the 'host' (individual) and is influenced by the 'environment' (community, culture, norms settings, politics, and values).

Albert Bandura

The Social Learning Theory of Albert Bandura emphasizes the importance of observing and modeling the behaviors, attitudes, and emotional reactions of others. Social Learning Theory explains human behavior in terms of continuous reciprocal interaction between cognitive, behavioral, and environmental influences.

Alternative Activities

This approach to substance abuse prevention is based on the assumption that involving high-risk youth in activities that are free of alcohol, tobacco, and other drugs will occupy their leisure time with prosocial activities and allow them to make friends with more social peers. This approach does NOT stand alone as an effective prevention strategy and should be paired with another CSAP strategy.

Analgesic

A drug that relieves pain by changing the perception of pain rather than by deadening the nerves of an anesthetic wound.

Archival Data

Data that already exists and that are maintained by an organization or entity. Examples include data from the Centers of Disease Control and Prevention, the National Institute on Drug Abuse, etc.

Assessment

A standardized tool to measure something specific, such as level of knowledge or attitudes and beliefs. We typically conduct a community needs assessment as the first step in understanding the substance misuse issues affecting a community.

Assimilation

A concept from Piaget's Cognitive Developmental Stages Theory. The process of adding new information to an existing schema.

ATOD

Alcohol, tobacco, and other drugs.

Basic Needs

From Maslow's Hierarchy of needs. These needs are primary and include: safety, sense of belonging, love, respect, and esteem. These needs must be met before progressing to 'growth.'

Best Practices
Prevention strategies, activities, or approaches that have been shown through research and evaluation to be effective in the prevention and/or delay of substance use or abuse.

Binge Drinking
When a man consumes five or more standard drinks in one sitting at least one day in the last 30 days. When a woman consumes four or more standard drinks in one sitting at least one day in the last 30 days.

CADCA
Community Anti-Drug Coalitions of America.

Capacity Building
The term 'capacity' refers to the various resource needed to implement prevention initiatives. 'Capacity Building' refers to increasing these resources and skills.

Cannabinols
The psychoactive cannabinoids of the cannabis plant.

Case Study
An in-depth study of an individual, group, or event, and represents a specific data collection method. Case studies are often subjective and cannot be used to make general statements about a population or circumstance.

Central Nervous System Depressant
A psychoactive drug, such as alcohol or an opiate that decreases the actions in the brain, resulting in depressed respiration, heart rate, muscle strength, and other functions.

Central Nervous System Stimulant
Any substance that forces the release of epinephrine and norepinephrine, that body's stimulants. They increase the electrical and chemical activity of the brain.

Channel
A component of the Process Model of Communication. The method by which information is communicated within the communication process.

Coalition
The formal name given to community mobilization types of efforts. A group of individuals and/or agencies agreeing to work together for a common purpose. Coalitions vary in formality, size, and composition.

Community Assessment
A systematic process for examining the current conditions and identifying the level of risk and protection within a community. It should also include the documentation of resources available in the community to address the problem areas. This term is often used interchangeably with needs assessment.

Community-Based Processes
Community-based processes are a CSAP 6 strategy. These strategies aim to enhance the ability of the community to more effectively provide prevention and treatment services for substance abuse. Services in this strategy include organizing, planning, and enhancing the efficiency and effectiveness of services implementation, interagency collaboration, coalition building, and networking.

Community Environment
The context where the substance uses issue occurs.

Community Mobilization
Community mobilization is a capacity-building process through which a community carries out and evaluates activities. Community mobilization empowers individuals and groups to take action to facilitate change based on the needs they have identified.

Community Norms
The attitudes toward policies about drug use and crime that a community holds. They are communicated in a variety of ways: through laws and written policies; through informal social practices; and through the expectations that parents and other members of the community have of young people.

Community Readiness
The extent to which a community is prepared to implement a substance abuse prevention program. The underlying premise of community readiness is changed in ATOD use cannot occur if there exists a high level of community denial about this problem.

Concrete Operations
A concept from Piaget's Cognitive Developmental Stages Theory, and last from ages 7 to 11. Piaget believed children in stage three are capable of symbolic or representational thought and can use logical operations, but they still cannot think abstractly. This is an important concept to remember when working with young audiences.

Continuum of Care
This continuum offers a comprehensive way of viewing the opportunities to intervene and address behavioral health problems. There are four primary components to the continuum: promotion, prevention, treatment, and recovery.

Copyright
Copyright is a legal device that provides the creator (art, music, document, literature) the right to control how the work is used.

CSAP
Center for Substance Abuse Prevention.

CSAP 6 Strategies
CSAP defined six broad prevention strategies: Information Dissemination, Prevention Education, Alternative Activities, Problem Identification and Referral, Community-Based Processes, and Environmental Approaches.

Cultural Competence
Cultural competence refers to the ability to interact effectively with individuals from different cultural backgrounds. It comprises four components: 1) Awareness of one's cultural world view; 2) Attitudes towards cultural differences; 3) Knowledge and awareness of different cultural practices, beliefs, and world views; and 4) Possessing cross-cultural skills.

Cultural Humility
Practicing cultural humility means reflecting on one's own culture and actively listening to the needs and experiences of those being served in the community.

Culture
The transfer of knowledge, experience, values, beliefs, ideas, attitudes, skills, tastes, and techniques that are shared and passed along from one member of the community to another member of the community.

Data Analysis
An examination of data to establish meaning and set priorities for community change.

Data Collection
Refers to the manner in which information is gathered in an evaluation. It can include interviews, surveys, focus groups, document reviews, and observations.

Deep Culture
Characteristics that cannot be seen by just looking at someone such as values or belief systems.

Delegator
Leadership style that focuses on assigning responsibilities to others and allowing them to follow through independently.

Developer
Leadership style with an emphasis on empowering others to make decisions.

Direct Cost
Those costs associated with the completion of the tasks, such as supplies, personnel, logistics (site costs, food, travel), and others.

Director
Leadership style characterized by independent decision making, delegation of explicit roles to team members, close supervision, and valuing those team members who align with their goals.

Disequilibrium
A concept from Piaget's Cognitive Developmental Stages Theory. An imbalance between assimilation and accommodation.

Environment
In the public health model, environment represents the broader context in which the 'agent' interacts with the 'host.' In AOD planning, the environment includes the community, culture, norms, laws, and regulations that affect the distribution and availability of the 'agent' (e.g., tobacco, alcohol, and other drugs). By changing the 'environment,' it is expected that changes will occur with the 'agent's' availability leading to reduced problems with the 'host' (individual).

Environmental Strategy
One of CSAP's Six Prevention Strategies. Environmental strategies are designed to address the complex set of factors in the environment, such as norms, media messages, laws and regulations, or accessibility. Environmental Prevention works to change the settings and messages that both directly and indirectly make drug use easy, appealing, attractive, and socially acceptable. This is done through a variety of approaches, including changes in public laws (conventional use permits), increased taxation on alcohol/tobacco products, countering media messages, reduce accessibility (e.g., server intervention, cutting off alcohol sales at sporting events), promoting nonuse behaviors (e.g., alcohol/drugfree community events, designated drivers, sober graduation).

Equilibration
A concept from Piaget's Cognitive Developmental Stages Theory. Describes the process of moving from disequilibrium to equilibrium.

Equilibrium
A concept from Piaget's Cognitive Developmental Stages Theory. Describes the cognitive balancing between assimilation and accommodation.

Erik Erikson
Created the Psychosocial Development Stages to describe a set of eight stages that an individual will experience in their lifetime. Erikson believed that personality development is predetermined and occurs in the order of these eight stages, from infancy to adulthood.

Ethics
The rules and standards governing professional conduct. We have six domains of ethical conduct: nondiscrimination, competence, integrity, nature of services, confidentiality, and ethical obligation to community and society.

External Assets
Created by Search Institute, External Assets are provided by the family, school, and community, and include support, empowerment, boundaries and expectations, and constructive use of time.

External Evaluation
Evaluation done by a consultant or organization not working on the prevention program.

Facilitator
A facilitator manages a group process to ensure: 1) a constructive discussion, 2) involvement of all members, and 3) team cohesiveness. A facilitator serves as a referee and does not take sides.

Feedback
A component of the Process Model of Communication. Verbal and nonverbal communication that occurs during and after a message has been sent.

Fidelity
This term applies to replicating a program model or strategy. To have 'fidelity,' the program needs to be implemented with the same specifications of the original program. Fidelity can be balanced with adaptation to meet local needs.

Focus Group
A group of people convened for the purpose of obtaining perceptions or opinions, suggesting ideas, or recommending actions. A focus group is a method of collecting information for the evaluation process.

Folx
Culturally inclusive spelling of the work 'folks' and it meant to be inclusive of all.

Formal Operations
A concept from Piaget's Cognitive Developmental Stages Theory, and last from ages 11 to 15. Children can think abstractly – or that they understand the distinction between reality and fantasy. This is defined as the point when an individual's cognitive structures have reached maturity.

Goal
Goal statements are broad, future-oriented action statements to be achieved by a program. Neither dates nor responsibilities are included.

Growth Needs
Includes the cognitive and self-actualization categories of Maslow's Hierarchy of Needs. Growth needs can be achieved after basic needs are met.

Guiding Principles
Findings of effective prevention programs as identified through research.

Hallucinogen
Substances that produce hallucinations, often used interchangeably with the terms psychedelic, psychotomimetic, and psychogenic.

Hearing
The physiological transference of sound waves into auditory nerve impulses, such as when a siren goes off or a phone rings.

Host
In the Public Health Model, the 'host' is the individual or person affected by the public health problem (e.g., the 'agent'; for prevention alcohol, tobacco, and other drugs).

Impacts
The ultimate effect of the program on the problem or condition that the program or activity was supposed to change. We typically look to make short- and long-term impacts on the community served. This term is often use interchangeable with outcomes.

Indicated
Those programs and strategies designed to target specific individuals at risk for substance abuse problems.

Indicator
A variable that relates directly to some part of a program goal or objective. Positive change on an indicator is presumed to show progress in accomplishing the larger program objective.

Indirect Cost
Costs to the agency not directly related to completing tasks, such as payroll, accounting, space, equipment, and general project administration.

Information Dissemination
One of CSAP's Six Prevention Strategies. Information Dissemination includes providing information and is characterized as one-way communication.

Information Overload
An overwhelming amount of information is conveyed at any one time.

Inhalant
Any substance that is vaporized, misted, or gaseous that is inhaled and absorbed through the capillaries in the alveoli of the lungs.

Input
A component in the logic model. These are the resources invested into the prevention program. Inputs can include money, staff, curriculum, etc.

Internal Asset
Created by Search Institute, Internal Assets are the values, commitments, competencies, and self-perceptions to be nurtured in every young person. They include a commitment to learning, positive values, social skills, and positive identity.

Internal Evaluation
A process of a quality review undertaken within an institution for its own ends (with or without the involvement of external peers).

IOM Model

The Institution of Medicine (IOM) developed an approach, that: 1) views prevention as part of an overall continuum of services, concluding with treatment; 2) identifies three levels of prevention: universal, selected, and indicated that refers to populations at varying levels of risk involving substances which in turn dictates that level and type of prevention services appropriate for the level of risk evident in the various population groupings.

Jean Piaget

Jean Piaget was a psychologist who studied how children learn and think. Jean Piaget's theory of cognitive development suggests that children move through four different stages of mental development: sensory-motor, preoperational, concrete operations, formal operations.

Key Informant Interview

A data collection method in which specific stakeholders are interviewed as a means of gathering information.

Listening

Not just hearing but also processing the information conveyed.

Lobbying

Taking a specific position on a specific piece of legislation or ballot proposition/initiative. There are specific restrictions concerning lobbying when a business is a 501c3.

Logic Model

Logic models show the underlying assumptions upon which an activity is expected to lead to a specific result. Logic models illustrate a sequence of cause and effect relationships. With a logic model, you are able to clearly connect your inputs, outputs, and outcomes.

Media Advocacy

The strategic use of media to advance a social or public policy initiative.

Media Literacy

The ability to access, analyze, and produce information for specific outcomes. The ability to 'read' and produce media messages.

Message

The information that the Sender is trying to communicate in the communication process.

Mission

A brief statement describing the purpose of organization or program.

Model Program

Prevention programs that have been rigorously evaluated and have repeatedly demonstrated positive outcomes.

Needs Assessment
A systematic process for examining the current conditions and identifying the level of risk and protection within a community. It should also include the documentation of resources available in the community to address the problem areas.

NIAAA
National Institute of Alcohol Abuse and Alcoholism.

NIDA
National Institute of Drug Abuse.

Noise
A component of the Process Model of Communication. Any impediment to a message's conveyance within the process model of communication.

Norms
A behavior or belief that is considered typical of a community. In prevention, work may be focused on changing negative norms, such as underage drinking, or it may be promoting positive norms, such as encouraging substance-free family gatherings.

Objective
Each goal has a set of objective statements. These are statements that, minimally, have four main qualities that distinguish them from goals or mission statements. Objectives should be SMART: 1) specific, 2) measurable, 3) achievable, and 4) timebound.

ONCDP
Office of National Drug Control Policy.

ORN
Opioid Response Network.

Outcome
Ways in which the participants of a prevention program could be expected to change at the conclusion of the program (e.g., increases in knowledge, changes in attitudes or behavior). We typically look to make short and long-term outcomes in the community served. This term is often used interchangeably with impact.

Output
The immediate products or activities of a program (e.g., the number of participants, number of hours of service, work accomplished). This term is often used interchangeably with activities.

Place
From the 4Ps of marketing. The communication channel for a social marketing campaign.

Posttest
A test or measurement taken after services or activities have ended. It is compared with the results of a pretest to show evidence of the effects or changes resulting from the services or activities being evaluated.

Praxis
The combination of theory and practice.

Preoperational Stage
A concept from Piaget's Cognitive Developmental Stages Theory, and last from ages 2 to 7. Children are capable of symbolic thought but cannot yet consolidate their thinking. This is thought of as a transitional phase where the learning of language is developed.

Pretest
A test or measurement is taken before services or activities begin. It is compared with the results of a posttest to show evidence of the effects of the services or activities being evaluated. A pretest can be used to obtain baseline data.

Prevalence
The proportion of a population with a specific characteristic. For example, the proportion of a population with a substance use disorder, or the proportion of the population who reports being drinking.

Prevention education
One of CSAP's Six Prevention Strategies. Prevention Education involves two-way communication, generally a facilitator/educator, and a group of learners (participants). Examples include classroom presentations, parenting and family management classes, and groups for children of substance abusers.

Price
From the 4Ps of marketing. What the consumer has to give up in order to achieve the benefits being offered in a social marketing campaign.

Primary Data
First-hand data collected by the organization.

Problem Identification and Referral
One of CSAP's Six Prevention Strategies. Problem Identification and Referral aims to identify those who have engaged in drug use in order to determine whether their behavior can be reversed through education (e.g., diversion programs) or whether they need a referral for a chemical dependency assessment. Examples include DUI education programs or Student Assistance Programs.

Problem Solver
Leadership style where group members are engaged in the problem-solving process and the leader makes decisions based on input from group members.

Process Evaluation
This form of evaluation assesses the extent to which a program is operating as it was intended. It typically assesses program activities' conformance to statutory and regulatory requirements, program design, and professional standards or customer expectations. Also known as an implementation evaluation and focuses on the outputs/activities for the program.

Process Model of Communication
This is a theory of communication with six component parts: sender, message, channel, receiver, feedback, and noise.

Product
From the 4Ps of marketing.

Promotion
From the 4Ps of marketing. The overall strategy or message that is used to persuade the target audience of a social marketing campaign.

Protective Factors
Protective factors, identified by Hawkins and Catalano, counter risks; the more protective factors are present, the less the risk. Protective factors fall into three basic categories: individual characteristics, bonding, and healthy beliefs, and clear standards.

Public Health Model
The Public Health Model of Prevention is based on the interaction of the 'host' (individual or person), the 'agent' (tobacco, alcohol, or other drugs), and the 'environment' (community setting, values, or policies).

Qualitative Data
Information that is difficult to measure, count, or express in numerical terms. Qualitative data may be presented in narrative form. Qualitative research typically uses observation, interviewing, open-ended responses, and document review to collect data.

Quantitative Data
Information that is reported in numerical forms such as substance use rates, number of people attending a program, or number of alcohol-related deaths. The strength of quantitative data is their use in testing hypotheses and determining the strength and direction of effects.

Receiver
A component of the Process Model of Communication. The individual(s) who take in the message from the Sender that was conveyed through the communication channel.

Resilience
Resilience is the ability of an individual to cope with or overcome the negative effects of 'risk' factors or to 'bounceback' from a problem (e.g., substance abuse).

Resilience Factors

Werner et al. contend that these are factors that protect or buffer people against social problems or risk factors. There are three clusters of factors present in resilient youths: 1) positive attitude or disposition, 2) healthy, strong relationship with a caring adult, and 3) having an external support system.

Risk Factors

Factors shown to increase the likelihood of adolescent substance use, teenage pregnancy, school dropout, youth violence, and delinquency. Risk factors occur in all areas of life: community, family, school, and individual/peer group. The more risk factors present, the greater the risk. The risk and protective factors theory are based on the work of David Hawkins, PhD, and Richard Catalano, PhD.

SAMHSA

Substance Abuse and Mental Health Services Administration.

Schema

A concept from Piaget's Cognitive Developmental Stages Theory. Describes the cognitive process of organizing information from the environment to make is easy to reference in the future. Schemata (plural for schema) are updated as the child ages and gains new knowledge.

Search Institute

The Search Institute created the Asset Developmental Model. Assets are relationships, opportunities, skills, values, and commitments children and adolescents need to grow up healthy, caring, and responsible. The research-based framework is organized into two types of assets: external and internal.

Secondary Data

Second-hand data collected by an outside source.

Sensory Motor Stage

A concept from Piaget's Cognitive Developmental Stages Theory, and last from ages birth to 2. Stage 1 is characterized by infants' discovery of their own bodies and all aspects related to them – you could describe an infant as thinking through touch.

Selective

Those programs and strategies designed to target specific groups at greater risk for AOD substance abuse problems (e.g., school dropouts, foster youths, incarcerated youths, children of alcoholics).

Sender

A component of the Process Model of Communication. This is the person conveying the information.

Social Development Strategy Model
Hawkins and Catalano's explanation of protective factors and healthy communities led to the social development theory which examines three broad domains: individual characteristics, healthy beliefs, and clear standards and bonding, and their respective protective factors.

Social Marketing
Environmental prevention strategy that presents messages to a population in a form similar to commercial messaging.

Social Norms Marketing
A strategy used to educate or communicate healthy behaviors as practiced by a majority of the public or selected group.

Standard Drink
12 fl oz of a 5% alcohol beer, 5 fl oz of 12% alcohol wine, 1.5 fl oz of 40% alcohol distilled spirit

Steroid
A steroid pharmacologically similar to testosterone that builds muscle and strength. It also induces male sexual characteristics.

Strategic Prevention Framework (SPF)
The SPF was developed by CSAP to provide the prevention field a logical framework for developing community-based prevention plans. It includes five distinct steps: 1) assessment; 2) capacity building; 3) planning; 4) implementation; and, 5) evaluation. SPF also has two cross-cutting concepts: sustainability and cultural competence.

Substance
Any psychoactive compound with the potential to cause health and social problems, and may cause substance use disorders.

Substance Misuse
Use of a psychoactive substance in a way that can cause harm, or use that is illegal (i.e., underage drinking).

Substance Use
Use of any psychoactive substances.

Surface culture
Characteristics such as race or ethnicity, which can be seen by simply looking at someone.

Survey
The collection of information from a common group through interviews, or the application of questionnaires to a representative sample of that group.

Theory
A formulation of relationships or principles of observed phenomena that has been verified, at least in part.

Universal
Those programs and strategies designed to target the entire population of a community (e.g., mass media campaigns).

Vision
What the program or organization hopes to accomplish in 5–10 years. This is the statement that describes how the community will look if you accomplish your goals.

Appendix A: History of Prevention Perspectives

Table A.1 This chart provides an overview of the history of prevention

Date	Perspective	Strategy
1950s	Drugs are a problem of the ghetto, used to escape pain and to avoid reality.	Scare tactics
Early 1960s	Drugs are used to escape pain and to avoid reality, but they're more than just a problem of the ghetto.	Scare tactics
Late 1960s	Drugs are used to intensify life, to have psychedelic experiences. Drug use is considered a national epidemic.	Scare tactics, information
Early 1970s	A variety of drugs are used for a variety of reasons: to speed up experiences, intensify experiences, escape, expand perceptions, relieve boredom, and conform to peer pressure.	Scare tactics, drug education, development of curricula
Mid 1970s	Users become more sophisticated and society develops an increasing tolerance of drug use.	Scare tactics, affective education, alternatives to drug use, development of curricula focused on communication, decision making, values, & self-esteem
Late 1970s to Mid 1980s	Parents begin to form organizations to combat drug abuse.	Scare tactics, affective education, alternatives to drug use, development of curricula focused on social skills, refusal skills, and parenting
Mid 1980s to Mid 1990s	Drug use is very complex.	Focus shift to parent, school, and community partnerships. Development of research-based curricula

(Continued)

Table A.1 (Continued)

Date	Perspective	Strategy
Mid 1990s to 2000	Substance misuse can be prevented through the dissemination of science-based programs which have been verified through an extensive evaluation.	Establishment of 'evidence-based' strategies and a national registry of effective programs. Additional focus on environmental approaches, evaluation, media, and cultural responsiveness
Mid 2000s to late 2010s	Drugs and drug use patterns are rapidly changing and require cross-agency cooperation. Resources must be maximized to create change at the community level.	Development of the Strategic Prevention Framework as the model planning tool. Formalization of funding, professional practices, and community-based initiatives.
Late 2010s to 2020s	Continued acknowledgment of the complex context that created substance use disorder.	Growth in the field to a focus on environmental strategies and the development of community-based processes. New shift to highlight disparities and health equity.

Index

Page numbers followed by "*f*" indicate figures; page numbers followed by "*t*" indicate tables

abstinence 43
academicians 42
accommodation 87
addiction, models of 51–2
addictive personality 51
advocacy tools, environmental
    change 78–9
agent, influencing 26, 26*f*
alternative activities, CSAP Six
    Strategies 29
anabolic steroids 46
andragogy 57
answers, Practice Questions 120;
    understanding 121–43
Anti-Drug Abuse Act of 1986 49
archival data 20, 21, 32
aspirin 46
assessing community readiness 16–19;
    confirmation/expansion 18–19; denial
    17; initiation 18; preparation 18;
    preplanning 17–18; professionalization
    19; stabilization/institutionalization
    18; vague awareness 17
assessment in SPF model 27
assets 83–4; external 84; internal 84
assimilation 87
attention 88
autonomy *vs.* shame 85

Bandura, Albert 88
Bandura's Social Learning Theory 88
basic needs 84
belongingness and love, Hierarchy of
    Needs Theory 84
best practices 23–4
biological model, addiction 52

biopsychosocial aspect, addiction 52
BIPOC. *See* Black, Indigenous, and
    People of Color (BIPOC)
Black, Indigenous, and People of Color
    (BIPOC) 49

Cannabis sativa 50
capacity in SPF model 27
Center for Substance Abuse Prevention
    (CSAP) Six Strategies 25, 28–9
central nervous system (CNS)
    depressants 48
central nervous system (CNS)
    stimulants 49
certification, prevention specialist 3–4
channel 55*f*, 56. *See also* communication
characterological/personality modal,
    addiction 51
coalition, effective 66–8; cohesion 67;
    diverse stakeholders 67–8; efficiency
    67; goal directedness 66–7; new skills
    68; opportunities for participation 68
coalition development 68–70
coalition management 70–1
cocaine 46
codeine 46, 47
cognitive, Hierarchy of Needs Theory 84
cognitive model, addiction 52
cognitive-developmental stages 87–8
cohesion 67
communication 54–64; group facilitation
    58–9; leadership styles 59–60; listening
    56–7; media advocacy 60–4; process
    model of 55–6, 55*f*; public speaking
    57–8; self-assessment 54–5, 54*t*; social

marketing 62–3; social norms
  marketing 63–4, 63*f*
Communities That Care (CTC) model
  25, 29–30; planning stages 30
community issue, prioritization 21
community mobilization 78
community needs assessment 19–21
community of focus 22–3
community organization 65–72;
  coalition, effective 66–8; coalition
  development 68–70; coalition
  management 70–1; community
  readiness 66; consensus, building 71–2;
  self-assessment 65–6
community organizing 77–8
community prevention board 30
community readiness 66
community resources/capacity,
  assessment 22
community-based processes, CSAP Six
  Strategies 29
comparison group 32
competencies, prevention specialist:
  Domain I: Planning and Evaluation
  15–35; Domain II: Prevention
  Education and Service Delivery 38–52;
  Domain III: Communication 54–64;
  Domain IV: Community Organization
  65–72; Domain V: Public Policy and
  Environmental Change 73–80;
  Domain VI: Professional Growth and
  Responsibility 81–101; Prevention
  Code of Ethics 90–2
Concrete Operations stage 87
conditioning model, addiction 52
confidentiality 97–8
confirmation/expansion stage 18–19
consensus, building 71–2
continuum of care 43–5, 44*f*
Controlled Substance Act (CSA) 45–7;
  Schedules 46–7
cough medicines 47
COVID-19 pandemic, social dimension
  and 99
creativity *vs.* stagnation 86–7
CSA. *See* Controlled Substance Act (CSA)
CSAP Six Strategies 25, 28–9
CTC model 29–30; planning stages 30
cultural adaptations 41–2
cultural competency 38–41; critical steps
  40–1; deep culture 40; defined 38–9; in
  SPF model 28; surface culture 40
culture 39; deep 40; surface 40

D.A.R.E. (Drug Resistance and
  Education) program 68
Darvon* 47
data: archival 20, 21, 32; primary 20, 21,
  32; qualitative 34; quantitative 34;
  statistical 61
data analysis 20
data collection 20; archival data 20, 21,
  32; options 32; primary data 20, 21, 32
data literacy 20
deep culture 40
delegator 60
denial stage 17
depressants, CNS 48
developer 60
Developmental Assets Model 83–4
developmental stages 87
director 59
disequilibrium 87
dispositional disease 52
dissemination of information, CSAP Six
  Strategies 28
diverse stakeholders 67–8
domains: Domain I: Planning and
  Evaluation 15–35; Domain II:
  Prevention Education and Service
  Delivery 38–52; Domain III:
  Communication 54–64; Domain IV:
  Community Organization 65–72;
  Domain V: Public Policy and
  Environmental Change 73–80;
  Domain VI: Professional Growth and
  Responsibility 81–101
'downers' 48
drug policies, history of 7–9
drug use, stigma of 9, 10*t*

economic stability, SDOH 10
education access and quality, SDOH 11
education modal, addiction 51
emotional wellness 99–100
environment, influencing 26–7, 26*f*
environmental approaches, CSAP Six
  Strategies 29
environmental change, tools of 76–9, 77*t*;
  advocacy tools 78–9; community
  mobilization 78; community
  organizing 77–8
environmental dimension, wellness 99
environmental strategies 74–6, 74*f*, 77*f*,
  85; use of media in supporting 79–80
epidemiology 61
equilibration 87

equilibrium 87
Erikson, Erik 85–7
Erikson's Psychosocial Development
    Stages 85–7
ethical dilemma 89
ethical obligations for community and
    society 98–9
evaluation: defined 30; methods and
    study design 32–5, 34*t*–35*t*; plan 30–5,
    33*t*, 34*t*–35*t*; questions 33*t*, 34*t*–35*t*;
    significance of 31; in SPF model 28;
    terms and concepts 31–2
expansion stage 18–19
external assets 84

facilitating effective meetings 70–1
facilitation 58–9
feedback 55*f*, 56
financial wellness 100–1
Formal Operations stage 87
'4Ps' of marketing 62–3
framing the issue 61

general systems 52
generativity *vs.* stagnation 86
goal directedness 66–7
group facilitation 58–9
growth needs 84
guiding principles 23–4

hallucinogens 50
health, social determinants of 10–11
health care access and quality, SDOH 11
hearing 56
heroin 46
Hierarchy of Needs Theory 84–5
higher needs 84
host, influencing 26, 26*f*
Human Development Theories 84–8;
    Cognitive-Developmental Stages 87–8;
    Hierarchy of Needs 84–5; Psychosocial
    Development Stages 85–7; Social
    Learning Theory 88
hydrocodone 46

IC&RC Standards 105–7
identity *vs.* role confusion 86
impact 32
implementation in SPF model 28
indicated prevention strategy 22–3
industry *vs.* inferiority 86
inhalants 50–1
initiation stage 18

initiative *vs.* guilt 85–6
integrity 92–4
intellectual wellness 101
internal assets 84
International Certification & Reciprocity
    Consortium 54, 88
intimacy *vs.* isolation 86

'Just Say NO!' Campaign 68

leadership styles 59–60
listening 56–7; *versus* hearing 56; noise
    and 57
lobbying 99
logic model 24–30; example 25*t*, 33*t*,
    34*t*–35*t*
LSD 46

marijuana 46
Maslow, Abraham 84
Maslow's Hierarchy of Needs 84–5
media: advocacy 60–4; in environmental
    strategies 79–80; gaining access to 61–2
media literacy 62
message 55–6, 55*f*.
    See also communication
methadone 46
methamphetamine 46
methaqualone 46
'mid-life crisis' 86
'misuse' (substance) 43
mobilize the community for action 19
modeled behavior 88
moral model, addiction 51
morphine 46
motivation 88
motor reproduction 88

narcotics 47–8
National Association of Prevention
    Professionals and Advocates 88
National Institute on Drug Abuse
    (NIDA) 23
nature of services 94–7
needs assessment 19–21; archival data,
    gathering 21; primary data, need for
    21; purpose and scope, defining 21
neighborhood and build environment,
    SDOH 11
new skills 68
NIDA. *See* National Institute on Drug
    Abuse (NIDA)
'no use' (substance) 43

noise: listening and 57; process model of communication 55*f*, 56; public speaking and 57–8
nondiscrimination 89–90

observational learning 88
occupational wellness 100
OTC. *See* over-the-counter (OTC) medicines
outcome evaluation 31–2
outcomes 32
outputs 32
over-the-counter (OTC) medicines 49

participation, coalition, opportunities for 68
phencyclidine (PCP) 46
PHM. *See* public health model (PHM)
physical wellness 100
Piaget, Jean 87–8
Piaget's Cognitive-Developmental Stages 87–8
place, in social marketing 62
planning and evaluation: assessing community readiness 16–19; community issue, prioritization 21; community of focus 22–3; 'guiding principles' and 'best practices' 23–4; logic model 24–30, 25*t*, 33*t*, 34*t*–35*t*; mobilize the community for action 19; needs assessment 19–21; program evaluation 30–5, 33*t*, 34*t*–35*t*; resource assessments 22; self-assessment 15–16, 15*t*–16*t*
planning in SPF model 28
planning models: Communities That Care (CTC) model 25, 29–30; CSAP Six Strategies 25, 28–9; public health model (PHM) 25, 26–7, 26*f*; strategic prevention framework (SPF) 25, 27–8, 27*f*
posttest, data collection 32
Practice Questions, Set 1 107–15; understanding the correct answer 121–35
Practice Questions, Set 2 115–19; understanding the correct answer 135–43
preamble 89
preoperational stage 87
preparation stage 18
preplanning stage 17–18

pretest, data collection 32
prevention, in continuum of care model 43, 44*f*, 45
Prevention Code of Ethics 88–99; preamble 89; principle 1: nondiscrimination 89–90; principle 2: competency 90–2; principle 3: integrity 92–4; principle 4: nature of services 94–7; principle 5: confidentiality 97–8; principle 6: ethical obligations for community and society 98–9
prevention education, CSAP Six Strategies 29
prevention education and service delivery 38–52; addiction, models of 51–2; cultural competency 38–41; self-assessment 38, 38*t*; substance use 43–51
prevention perspectives, history of 159*t*–160*t*
prevention planning 23–4
prevention practice, social justice and 11–12
prevention program delivery 24
prevention specialist certification 3–4
Prevention Specialist Job Task Analysis 54
Prevention Think Tank 88
Prevention Think Tank Code 89
price, in social marketing 62
primary data: collection 20, 21, 32; need for 21
principles, Prevention Code of Ethics: competency 90–2; confidentiality 97–8; defined 89; ethical obligations for community and society 98–9; integrity 92–4; nature of services 94–7; nondiscrimination 89–90
prioritization models 21
problem identification and referral, CSAP Six Strategies 29
problem solver 59–60
process evaluation 31
product, in social marketing 62
professional growth and responsibility: Human Development Theories 84–8; personal wellness 99–101; Prevention Code of Ethics 88–99; self-assessment 81, 81*t*; theoretical models 82–4
professionalization: benefits of 4–5; certification, requirement of 3–4; stage 19
program evaluation 30–5, 33*t*, 34*t*–35*t*
program fidelity 41

promotion: in continuum of care model
43, 44*f*; in social marketing 63
promotion, in social marketing 63
psychological model, addiction 52
Psychosocial Development Stages 85–7
public health model (PHM) 25, 26–7,
26*f*, 52
public policy and environmental change
73–80; environmental strategies 74–6,
74*f*, 77*f*; self-assessment 73*t*; tools of
environmental change 76–9, 77*t*; use of
media 79–80
public speaking 57–8.
See also communication

qualitative data 34
quantitative data 34
questions: Practice Questions, Set 1
107–15; Practice Questions, Set 2
115–19; understanding the correct
answer 121–35

Reagan, Nancy 68
receiver 55*f*, 56. *See also* communication
recovery, in continuum of care model
44*f*, 45
recycling 100
research: cultural adaptations 42; media
advocacy 60–1
resiliency approach 83
resource assessments 22
respect and esteem, Hierarchy of Needs
Theory 84
retention 88
risk and protective factors 23
risk and protective factors theory 82

safety, Hierarchy of Needs Theory 84
SBIRT. *See* Screening, Brief Intervention,
and Referral to Treatment (SBIRT)
Schedule I drug 46
Schedule II drug 46
Schedule III drug 46–7
Schedule IV drug 47
Schedule V drug 47
schema 87
Screening, Brief Intervention, and
Referral to Treatment (SBIRT) 29
SDOH. *See* social determinants of health
(SDOH)
SDS. *See* Social Development
Strategy (SDS)
selective prevention strategy 22

self-actualization, Hierarchy of Needs
Theory 84
self-assessment: Domain I: Planning and
Evaluation 15–16, 15*t*–16*t*; Domain II:
Prevention Education and Service
Delivery 38, 38*t*; Domain III:
Communication 54–64; Domain IV:
Community Organization 65–6;
Domain V: Public Policy and
Environmental Change 73, 73*t*;
Domain VI: Professional Growth and
Responsibility 81, 81*t*
sender 55, 55*f*. *See also* communication
sensory-motor stage 87
social and community context, SDOH 11
social determinants of health (SDOH)
10–11
Social Development Strategy (SDS) 30
social justice, prevention practice and
11–12
social learning model, addiction 52
Social Learning Theory 88
social marketing 62–3.
See also communication; '4Ps' of
marketing 62–3
social norms marketing 63–4, 63*f*
social wellness 99
sociocultural context: prevention practice
6–12; substance use 6
sociocultural model, addiction 52
SPF. *See* strategic prevention
framework (SPF)
spiritual modal, addiction 51
spiritual wellness 101
statistical data 61
steroids 50
stimulants, CNS 49
strategic prevention framework (SPF) 25,
27–8, 27*f*
substance: categories of 47–51;
Controlled Substance Act (CSA) 45–7;
Schedules, CSA 46–7; 'use' 43
Substance Abuse and Mental Health
Services Administration 27
substance use: sociocultural context 6;
stigma of 9, 10*t*
substance use disorder 43
surface culture 40
surveys 34
sustainability in SPF model 28

temperance modal, addiction 51
temperance movement 51

theoretical models 82–4; Developmental Assets Model 83–4; resiliency approach 83; risk and protective factors theory 82
treatment, in continuum of care model 44*f*, 45
trust *vs.* mistrust 85
Tylenol* 46

United States: drug policies, history of 7–9
universal prevention strategies 22
'uppers' 49
'use' (substance) 43

vague awareness stage 17
Valium* 47
values 88–9

'War on Drugs' 48
wellness, dimensions of 99–101; emotional 99–100; environmental 100; financial 100–1; intellectual 101; occupational 100; physical 100; social 99–100; spiritual 101

Xanax* 47